FIGHT BACK:
BEAT THE CORONAVIRUS

FIGHT BACK:

BEAT THE CORONAVIRUS

By Dr. Chauncey W. Crandall IV, M.D.,
and Charlotte Libov

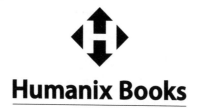

Humanix Books

Humanix Books, P.O. Box 20989, West Palm Beach, FL 33416, USA
www.humanixbooks.com | info@humanixbooks.com

Disclaimer: The information presented in this book is not specific medical advice for any individual and should not substitute medical advice from a health professional. If you have (or think you may have) a medical problem, speak to your doctor or a health professional immediately about your risk and possible treatments. Do not engage in any care or treatment without consulting a medical professional.

ISBN: 9781630061692 (Paperback)
ISBN: 9781630061708 (E-book)

Printed in the United States of America
10   9   8   7   6   5   4   3   2   1

To my colleagues, the physicians and nurses on the front line of battle of the coronavirus 19 pandemic that has stopped the world.

Also to my patients the Lord has entrusted to me.

My prayer is always for your protection and perfect health.

May God keep you safe.

—Dr. Chauncey Crandall

To the memory of my aunt Sylvia, who was paralyzed in the Spanish flu pandemic, and to my mother, Henny Libov, who devoted her life to her care.

—Charlotte Libov

His faithfulness will be a protective shield.
You will not fear the terror of the night,
the arrow that flies by day,

the plague that stalks in darkness,
or the pestilence that ravages at noon.

Though a thousand fall at your side
and ten thousand at your right hand,
the pestilence will not reach you.

—Psalm 91

CONTENTS

Part One:
COVID-19: What You Need to Know

Part Two:
How to Prevent COVID-19

Part Three:
Get Healthy to Fight COVID-19

Part Four:
Treating and Protecting against COVID-19

A NOTE FROM DR. CRANDALL

When I awakened on January 21, 2020, there was no hint of the nightmare to come. But the first case of an unknown illness had just been confirmed in Washington state, and the 2019 novel coronavirus, or coronavirus 2019 (COVID-19), had begun silently creeping into the United States. Fewer than three months later, all of our fifty states would be under a disaster declaration for the first time in U.S. history!

How could this happen? How could a microscopic viral pathogen bring down not only our economy but that of other great countries in the world?

Unlike some others, I have seen other pandemics up close. I have been involved in fighting epidemics throughout my career, including AIDS, malaria, dysentery, and cholera.

Prior to becoming a cardiologist, I trained to become an anthropologist, and I learned to appreciate that there is more than Western medicine, that the medical systems created by ancient cultures have much to teach us.

One thing that has perplexed scientists since the world first learned of COVID-19 is the mystery of how this pathogen can cause such wildly varying results. It's puzzling how some people don't even get symptoms, others survive it relatively unscathed, and yet in some people, it kills.

I can come to only one conclusion—our best defense against COVID-19 is to prevail over this virus by becoming stronger and healthier and by strengthening our immune system so that can fight back against it.

Throughout this book, I will give you many strategies to use in fighting COVID-19, and as this is a formidable virus, I want you to pay attention to all of them.

But pay special attention to the chapters in part 3 on immunity, because I believe that within the immune system lies the secret to how you can personally fight back against COVID-19.

* * *

We must remember we are at war now with an invisible enemy, and Winston Churchill's statement is just as pertinent now as it was during World War II:

"We shall fight on the beaches, we shall fight on the landing grounds, we shall fight in the fields and in the streets, we shall fight in the hills; we shall never surrender!"

The Arrival of COVID-19

The first cluster of cases caused by coronavirus 19 was announced by China on December 31, and less than a month later, a thirty-five-year-old man in Snohomish County, Washington, became the first COVID-19 case to be confirmed in the United States.

At the very same time, coronavirus 19, the virus that causes the disease COVID-19, was spreading rapidly through Asia, and then Europe, and eventually to all corners of the globe. The outbreak was so massive that on March 11, the World Health Organization (WHO) proclaimed it to be a pandemic, one of those rare diseases whose scale is so enormous that it sweeps across all international borders, affecting the whole world.

By the time we awakened on April 12, Easter Sunday, most of America had self-isolated to try to halt the spread of COVID-19; almost all of our churches and synagogues were closed, our hotels empty, and our cafés and restaurants shuttered. Nursing homes were barred to visitors to attempt to stem the tragic outbreaks there; most of our parks, beaches, and playgrounds were barricaded, and where massive outbreaks had occurred, convention centers and stadiums had been transformed into field hospitals.

By the end of April, just one hundred days since that first U.S. case was confirmed, our streets were still empty; even bustling thoroughfares like New York's Fifth Avenue. Las Vegas was a ghost town, its casinos closed, its shows canceled, and its famous strip deserted.

What happened was something that almost none of us had ever seen in our lifetimes or could have ever imagined; the United States of America had been shut down, closed to business because of a microscopic, invisible, viral pathogen.

As this book goes to press, America is emerging from lockdown, but even as this is happening, there are fears of a second wave of the disease expected to come in the fall and possibly beyond that as well. Remember, until we have a vaccine, COVID-19 remains an invisible enemy, a ticking time bomb!

Note: As we went to press, the information in this book was as current as possible, but scientists are working at breakneck speed to find answers and new treatments for COVID-19, so new information is constantly emerging. For updates, please go to the Newsmax Coronavirus Resource Page link: https://www.newsmax.com/coronavirus.

PART ONE

COVID-19:
What You Need to Know

CHAPTER 1

Why COVID-19 Is Worse
Than the Flu

The flu has been around for centuries, during which time we humans have built up a "herd" immunity, meaning that our immune systems have learned to mount at least some response to it, and have also developed a vaccination for those who wish to take it.

COVID-19 is different. It is caused by a new strain of the coronavirus that we have never seen before, so as of now, we have no immunity to it, there is no vaccine, and there is no cure.

Since its discovery last December, it's also becoming obvious that the coronavirus is significantly more lethal than seasonal flu and has seeded the most disruptive pandemic in one hundred years.

New serological data just coming in suggests that infections outnumber confirmed coronavirus cases by a factor of ten or more, since many people don't experience symptoms, so they aren't tested or counted in the case tally. But infectious disease specialists know that a disease with a small mortality rate can cause soaring death tolls when it infects millions of people, which is happening with COVID-19.

COVID-19 spreads like wildfire. Somewhere between 40 and 70 percent of the world's population can be infected in the next couple of years if there's no vaccine or no steps are taken to limit its spread.

Also, even though its termed a respiratory disease, it's becoming obvious that COVID-19 damages the whole body.

The coronavirus enters the body through the eyes, nose, or mouth and latches onto certain cells covered with an ACE2 enzyme receptor.

For most people, that seems to be where it stays, causing only mild symptoms or none at all.

But in one out of every six cases, it travels farther down the body into the lungs and into the bloodstream, and from there, it can enter and invade other organs, resulting in a wide variety of damage.

The coronavirus can infiltrate both the heart and the lungs because they each contain cells covered with the same ACE2 enzyme receptor.

The coronavirus can also head for other organs that contain these enzyme receptors as well, including the small and large intestines, the liver, and the kidneys. Just recently these receptors have been found lining cells of the nose.

While some of the organ damage is caused by the virus's invasion, along with the inflammation that results, the deadliest cases are those in which the immune system, sensing its widespread damage, suddenly goes into abnormal chaotic overdrive, creating a condition called a cytokine storm, which is much like aggressive friendly fire in the heat of battle.

When this happens, the body releases immune cells and proteins into the bloodstream, which then attack healthy tissues in the body. While such a response only occurs in a small percentage of cases, it can lead to organ shutdown and death.

The Lungs

When the coronavirus targets the lungs, it causes shortness of breath, which sometimes rapidly develops into acute respiratory distress syndrome, or ARDS. This condition causes massive fluid buildup in the lungs, preventing oxygen from getting to the rest of the body. This lack of oxygen can damage the body's other organ systems, causing them to shut down, and resulting in death.

The Heart

Research out of China shows not only that the virus damaged the lungs but that nearly 20 percent of people hospitalized with COVID-19 also suffered serious cardiac injury and were at higher risk of dying.

Such cardiac problems included sudden heart attacks, a serious heart condition known as myocarditis, and irregular heartbeat rhythms.

Initially, doctors chalked these problems up to the inflammatory effects of the virus, along with respiratory distress caused by pneumonia and ARDS, but they are now seeing other types of heart damage as well, leading them to believe the virus may injure the heart directly.

The Brain

Researchers are also concerned about mounting evidence that the coronavirus may attack the brain, causing neurological damage and even strokes.

In China, doctors reported a study that 30 percent of COVID-19 patients developed a wide array of neurological problems, including headache; dizziness; impaired consciousness; acute cerebrovascular disease, including epilepsy; and peripheral symptoms, including decreased appetite, taste, and smell.

In New York, doctors reported in the *New England Journal of Medicine* on a small number of apparently healthy younger people, who had suffered strokes and tested positive for COVID-19. The strokes occurred in the brain and were very unusual in people under the age of fifty. This has led doctors in New York to suspect that COVID-19 is causing a clotting problem that is leading to the strokes.

The paper also noted that in China, there was an approximate 5 percent incidence of strokes seen in COVID-19 patients, and strokes were also associated with the 2004 Singapore outbreak of severe acute respiratory syndrome (SARS), which is caused by a related type of coronavirus.

An article in *The New York Times* titled "Coronavirus May Pose a New Risk to Younger Patients: Strokes" (May 14, 2020) underscores this connection to COVID-19.

COVID-19 in Children and Teens

When COVID-19 first appeared in the United States, it was assumed that although children could contract and also spread the virus, they did not become seriously ill. But there are recent reports of children and teenagers becoming very sick with an inflammatory syndrome that may be linked to the virus. This new condition, considered rare, is called pediatric multisystem inflammatory syndrome, and it resembles Kawasaki disease, an acute illness in children.

This syndrome is considered very rare, and children with it have been hospitalized but have generally recovered.

While no link has been firmly established yet between this illness and COVID-19, it is being reported in areas where there have been large outbreaks of the virus, including in the United States, the United Kingdom, and other European countries.

A definitive list of symptoms is being compiled, but Kawasaki disease produces a persistent fever (102.2° Fahrenheit or higher), swollen neck glands, cracked lips, swelling in the hands and feet, and reddened eyes.

CHAPTER 2

Who Is at Risk?

*E*veryone is at risk of getting sick from COVID-19 because we have no built-in immunity to it. However, there are some groups within the population who are at even higher risk of developing serious complications from COVID-19. But remember, no one is immune from COVID-19.

That said, if you are in one of these categories, you are at high risk for developing complications from COVID-19 or even dying. Note that what many of these conditions have in common is a suppressed immune system. Having a strong immune system can help reduce your risk of infection from many viruses, including COVID-19.

Remember, if you are at risk for COVID-19, always talk to your doctor first to make sure the recommendations in this book are right for you.

Who Is at Highest Risk for Severe Complications for COVID-19

This list of risk factors is a long one, but a new British study called the International Severe Acute Respiratory and Emerging Infection Consortium (ISARIC) that surveyed seventeen thousand hospitalized coronavirus patients gives us the best understanding of who is actually at high risk.

The study, which analyzed patient data from February 2020 through April 2020, showed that the virus is virulent and quite often deadly. The study also found that certain preexisting conditions raise the risk of both complications and death.

Mortality rates for those hospitalized were high, with 33 percent of those admitted to a hospital for the virus dying. The mortality rates rose as patients developed complications, with 45 percent placed in intensive care units (ICUs) dying. Similarly, the study found that 53 percent of ICU patients placed on ventilators also died.

The study found the risk factors that raised the likelihood of dying were dementia (39 percent), obesity (37 percent), and heart disease (31 percent).

Metabolic Syndrome

The ISARIC study noted that patients who were hospitalized had certain preexisting conditions, including obesity, heart disease, and diabetes. Such conditions are often associated with the "metabolic syndrome" that afflicts one-third of adult Americans.

In fact, metabolic syndrome conditions skyrocket your risk of COVID-19 complications significantly more than if each condition was added singly. People with metabolic syndrome have two or more of the following conditions: obesity, high blood pressure, diabetes, high triglycerides, and low HDL cholesterol, the "good" cholesterol.

The ISARIC study found that of those hospitalized for the virus, 29 percent suffered from chronic heart disease, 19 percent had diabetes, 19 percent had pulmonary disease (not including asthma), and 14 percent had asthma.

Researchers who did a meta-analysis on studies in China involving 46,246 patients noted that, historically, they have fared worse in the viral pandemics preceding this one, mainly severe acute respiratory syndrome (SARS) and Middle East respiratory syndrome (MERS).

And COVID-19 is not shaping up to be an exception according to a study done in India, which found a death rate of nearly 50 percent for patients that had high blood pressure, diabetes, and heart disease.

Metabolic syndrome is seen as a disease largely caused by lifestyle, particularly eating too much and exercising too little. The good news is that you can take steps to reduce the severity of metabolic syndrome in your life, thereby reducing the risk due to exposure to the virus.

It is also important to remember that most of the conditions included in metabolic syndrome will weaken your immune system, so boosting your immune system is critically important to put you in the best position to fight back against COVID-19.

Now let's take a closer look at the risk factors that are more likely to make COVID-19 worse and also what steps to take to reduce these risks.

Risk Factors for COVID-19

- being age sixty-five and over
- high blood pressure
- obesity
- diabetes
- chronic lung diseases (chronic obstructive pulmonary disease [COPD] and asthma)
- cardiovascular disease, including heart disease and atrial fibrillation
- kidney disease
- immunosuppression
- cancer and being a cancer survivor

Age Sixty-Five and Over

Since the coronavirus was first identified, one fact has stood out consistently: those people who become most seriously ill have been age sixty-five and older. If you're in this age group, protecting against COVID-19 becomes extra important. If you're age eighty-five and older, you have the highest risk of dying of the disease.

Recommendations:

- Follow the recommendations on wearing a mask and social distancing outlined elsewhere in this book.
- If you work, ask your employer whether you can work from home.
- During the pandemic, restaurants were closed. When you go to them after they've reopened, give yourself some distance in seating and steer clear of any buffets to minimize the possibility of contamination.
- Make use of the special "Senior Hours" at supermarkets and other stores, both for those age sixty-five and older and for those at risk with other health conditions outlined here.
- At times when the virus is spreading, steer clear of crowds, including those at "senior" events, especially if people are not wearing masks or taking precautions.

- If meals are an issue, ask your municipality if you qualify for "Meals on Wheels."
- Avoid mass transit; if you don't drive, ask your local municipality or senior center about vans or smaller buses and make sure drivers are taking precautions.

High Blood Pressure

In every country hit by the virus, one thing also stands out—having high blood pressure, or hypertension, also puts you at the highest risk for being hospitalized or dying if you get COVID-19.

But why is this so? One possible explanation is that having high blood pressure weakens the heart and makes people with it more vulnerable to pulmonary problems.

But there is another possible reason, and this has to do with how high blood pressure is treated. There is a controversy surrounding the common high blood pressure drugs called ACE inhibitors and angiotensin receptor blockers (ARBs).

Here's the issue: When the coronavirus enters the body, it finds cells lined with ACE2 receptors to replicate and destroy. ACE inhibitors and ARBs, which are high blood pressure medications, can upgrade the number of ACE2 receptor sites, giving the virus more points in the body to attack and potentially making the disease outcome and course more severe and lethal.

Several medical associations, including the American College of Cardiology and the American Heart Association, contend that these concerns are unproven and people should continue to take these drugs as prescribed. There is also a contention that these drugs may actually help treat COVID-19 by providing decoy cells for the virus to attack.

But as there are other drugs that can lower blood pressure, most notably calcium channel blockers and beta-blockers, it seems to make sense to ask your doctor if one of these drugs would work just as well for you. Of course, never discontinue taking prescription drugs or change them without your doctor's approval.

Recommendations:
- Make sure you have a thirty-day supply of your medication.
- Keep your blood pressure under control.
- Be careful of certain medications, like NSAIDs, and certain decongestants, which can raise blood pressure, as can some drugs

that treat mental health conditions, corticosteroids, oral birth control, medications that suppress the immune system, some cancer medications, over-the-counter drugs, and supplements.

- Limit your intake of caffeine, certain teas, and energy drinks that have stimulants that can raise blood pressure. The candy licorice can do this as well.
- Buy a home blood pressure monitor and use it to keep an eye on your blood pressure.
- Ask about using telemedicine for follow-up visits.

Diabetes

Researchers in China found that people with diabetes had three times the death rates as those without diabetes, and studies in other countries have found this as well. People with diabetes have also been found to be at greater risk if they take ACE inhibitors or ARBs, and the possible reason can be found above in this chapter, so talk to your doctor if you take these medications. Also, people with type 2 diabetes (the most common form) may have an altered immune response, and those with type 1 diabetes have a tendency to develop a condition known as diabetic ketoacidosis. Diabetic ketoacidosis can result in severe dehydration, worsening other serious complications of COVID-19.

Recommendations:

- Make sure you have a thirty-day supply of your medication.
- Maintain tight blood sugar control to help reduce the risk of infections and complications.
- Keep a ninety-day supply of diabetes supplies, medications, and insulin (if you use it) on hand.
- Consider using telemedicine for follow-up doctor's visits.

Obesity

Obesity is a major factor for serious complications of COVID-19, no matter what age the person is.

A person whose body mass index, or BMI, is thirty or more is considered obese. BMI is based on a formula that divides a person's weight in kilograms by their height in meters.

According to the Centers for Disease Control and Prevention (CDC), nearly half (48.3 percent) of adults hospitalized in the United

States with COVID-19 were obese and were also most likely to require intensive care or die. Although these figures were based on people age sixty-five and older, other studies have found this to be true for younger people as well.

Exactly why obesity raises risk is unknown, but one possible explanation is that abdominal obesity, the pattern found mostly in men, may compress the diaphragm, lungs, and chest area. This makes breathing more difficult, especially when these individuals are sick.

Recommendations:
- Use COVID-19 as extra motivation to lose weight.
- See the chapter on what to eat (chapter 17) as well as the chapters on sleep (chapter 16), exercise (chapter 19), and stress reduction (chapter 20), as people under stress or those who are sleep deprived tend to eat more and gain weight.

Chronic Obstructive Pulmonary Disease

Chronic obstructive pulmonary disease, or COPD, is the umbrella term used to encompass the serious lung conditions of emphysema and chronic bronchitis. Studies find that people with COPD are at a fivefold risk for being hospitalized with severe COVID-19 and are also at greater risk of dying.

Recommendations:
- Make sure you have a thirty-day supply of your medication.
- If you use oxygen, contact your supplier to find out what to do in the event there is a COVID-19 outbreak in your area.
- People with COPD are at increased risk for severe complications from seasonal flu and pneumonia, so contact your physician if you are having symptoms of an upper respiratory infection.
- Ask about using telemedicine for follow-up visits.

Asthma

Early research on COVID-19 assumed that people with asthma would be at risk for complications because this disease constricts the airwaves, making it difficult to breathe. Later research finds that people with mild asthma are not at higher risk, but there is still a concern about those with moderate and severe asthmatic conditions.

Recommendations
- Follow your usual plan to keep your asthma under control.
- Make sure you have a thirty-day supply of your medication.
- Continue your current medications, including any with steroids. Although steroids can suppress the immune system, don't stop taking them without your doctor's approval.
- Avoid your asthma triggers. Also, asthma can be triggered by anxiety, and certainly the COVID-19 pandemic has caused anxiety, as are likely any reoccurrences of virus spread. Take care of your emotional health.
- Ask about using telemedicine for follow-up visits.

Heart Disease

People with heart disease are at an increased risk of serious complications from COVID-19 and also are more likely to die from it; they are at 10.5 percent increased risk of dying compared to 2.3 percent for people who do not have underlying health conditions, Chinese researchers say.

People with the following heart conditions are at highest risk, the European Society of Cardiology says:

- Heart failure, a condition in which the heart becomes weakened and doesn't pump blood effectively.
- Dilated cardiomyopathy, a disorder in which the heart's chambers become enlarged and cannot pump blood effectively.
- Advanced forms of arrhythmogenic right ventricular cardiomyopathy.
- Congenital cyanotic heart disease, which are types of heart problems that occur before birth and result in low blood oxygen levels.
- Obstructive hypertrophic cardiomyopathy.
- People who have undergone heart transplants are put on immunosuppressive drugs to keep their bodies from rejecting their new organs. This makes them more vulnerable to infections, including COVID-19.

Recommendations:
- Make sure all your vaccinations are up to date, including your pneumonia shot.

- Make sure you have a thirty-day supply of your medication.
- Ask about using telemedicine for follow-up visits.
- Review the information on ACE inhibitors and ARBs covered in the section in this chapter on high blood pressure and discuss with your doctor if you are taking any of these medications.
- Even during a COVID-19 outbreak, if you are experiencing any symptoms that can be heart-related, call 911. Such symptoms include the following:
  ◇ chest pain or discomfort
  ◇ difficulty breathing
  ◇ weakness
  ◇ shortness of breath
  ◇ fainting
  ◇ confusion

People with Weakened Immune Systems

Conditions that suppress the immune system include AIDS, HIV, and immune deficiency. People who have undergone bone marrow or organ transplants have weakened immune systems as well. The prolonged use of corticosteroids and TNF inhibitors, like adalimumab (Humira) and infliximab (Remicade), also weaken the immune system.

Recommendations:
- Discuss your condition with your doctor.
- Ask about using telemedicine for follow-up visits.

Kidney Disease

Serious kidney disease weakens the immune system, putting people at risk for infections, and this is even more true for those on dialysis. People with a kidney transplant need to take antirejection drugs, which work by suppressing the immune system.

Recommendations:
- If you have moderate or severe chronic kidney disease (stages 3–5), you should practice social distancing but also ask your doctor if you need to isolate yourself during times of COVID-19 spread. The more advanced your kidney disease, the stricter you need to be about avoiding interaction with others.

- If you're on dialysis, discuss your schedule with your treatment team. You also may be advised by your physician to isolate yourself from others to avoid getting infected.
- Ask about using telemedicine for follow-up visits.

Cancer and Cancer Survivors

Cancer patients—especially those with blood and lung cancers or malignancies that have spread throughout the body—have three times the risk of death or severe complications from COVID-19 compared to people who don't have cancer, a large, multihospital study in China finds. Also, many cancer treatments suppress the immune system, which makes contracting infections, including COVID-19, more likely. These treatments include chemotherapy, radiation, and CART cell therapy, which suppress the body's immune system.

Recommendations:

- Make sure you have a thirty-day supply of your medications on hand.
- Contact your doctor several days before a scheduled appointment to make sure the office is open.
- Ask about using telemedicine for follow-up visits.

CHAPTER 3

Symptoms

COVID-19 is the highly infectious respiratory viral disease caused by a new coronavirus that was first identified in China in December 2019 and has since spread to all corners of the world.

One of the things that sets COVID-19 apart from other respiratory diseases is the wide variety of symptoms, and it's a list that keeps getting lengthier the more we learn about the coronavirus.

People with COVID-19 have reported a wide range of symptoms and have experienced them in gradations ranging from mild to severe. Symptoms may appear two to fourteen days after exposure, which is a far longer time span than what happens with seasonal influenza.

The Centers for Disease Control and Prevention (CDC) recently expanded its official list of COVID-19 symptoms from six to nine, an indication of how quickly knowledge about this disease changes. This is important because these are the symptoms that a health care official will be looking for if you need them to obtain a diagnostic test.

It is estimated that up to 50 percent of those with COVID-19 don't develop symptoms during the first few days, and some people experience none. You don't need to have symptoms of COVID-19 to spread the disease to others.

Symptoms of COVID-19

Fever

A fever is a sign of inflammation, and as we learned from China with all the photos of everyone having their temperature taken, this has been considered a hallmark of the disease.

But although a fever was presented as the main symptom of the disease, a recent study in the *Journal of the American Medical Association* on people with COVID-19 who were the sickest in New York City found that two-thirds of these patients did not present with a fever at all.

Regarding fever, the CDC considers a fever to be 100.4° Fahrenheit, but it also considers it to be a fever when someone feels hot to the touch, has previously reported feeling feverish, or is flushed or glassy-eyed.

If you do have a fever, consider that this likely could be a symptom of COVID-19. If you don't have a fever but do have other symptoms, don't rule this viral disease out either.

Cough
A dry cough was also associated with COVID-19 from the start, but some studies have found that coughing blood may also occur in a small number of cases. Although this may be frightening, it isn't necessarily a sign of a worsening condition, as this can be due to many causes, including airway inflammation.

Shortness of Breath or Difficulty Breathing
Because there has been a lot of focus on patients with serious cases of COVID-19 pictured in the ICU, struggling for breath, this has become the image that many people think about when they think of this disease. This can be a serious symptom, but it also may not be.

Chills
Aches and chills can be symptoms of many illnesses, including the flu, but according to a World Health Organization (WHO) study, only about 11 percent of COVID-19 patients develop chills.

Repeated Shaking with Chills
Also known as the "rigors," this is a reaction that can come on during a viral infection, when viruses or bacteria are released into the bloodstream, and can even make teeth chatter. This symptom has been observed in COVID-19.

Muscle Pain
According to a WHO study, 14 percent of people with COVID-19 complain of muscle aches.

Headache

Although headache isn't considered a common symptom of COVID-19, studies show that about 14 percent of people do experience it, about the same percentage that experience muscle pain.

Sore Throat

The coronavirus attacks the upper respiratory tract, so it's logical that a sore throat is one of the symptoms. However, a sore throat can also be a sign of a cold or even seasonal allergies, so unless you're suffering from other COVID-19 symptoms, you may just have one of these less serious conditions.

New Loss of Smell and Taste

In the beginning, when reports of this symptom surfaced, they were initially just thought of as anecdotal, but now studies find that the loss of smell and taste is not uncommon early in COVID-19 cases.

Also, a study published in the *Forum of Allergy and Rhinology* in April finds that these symptoms are more common in people whose cases of COVID-19 turn out to be mild. The senses of taste and smell also return in about two to four weeks after the patient has recovered.

Additional COVID-19 Symptoms

These are symptoms that research has indicated sometimes occur with COVID-19, but they are as yet on the CDC's list.

Nasal Congestion or Runny Nose

Nasal congestion and having a runny nose were originally reported as a way to distinguish COVID-19 from a cold or allergies, but these symptoms have been observed in virus patients as well.

Fatigue

Fatigue doesn't usually occur alone, but it can be suggestive of COVID-19 if other disease symptoms are present.

Digestive Symptoms

Although upper respiratory symptoms were the first noted with COVID-19, a study published in the *American Journal of Gastroenterology* found that of 206 patients with mild COVID-19, one-quarter had digestive symptoms only, 69 had both digestive and respiratory symptoms, and 89 had respiratory symptoms alone. Digestive symptoms included lack of appetite, diarrhea, nausea, and vomiting.

Neurological Symptoms

Since COVID-19 was first discovered in China, it's been found that the disease can cause neurological symptoms. In one of the early China studies, researchers looked at 224 patients and discovered that nearly half with severe cases had neurological issues, including dizziness, headaches, and impaired consciousness. They still don't know whether this is due to the inflammation the virus causes or whether the virus can pass through the blood-brain barrier and attack the brain directly.

Pink Eye

"Pink eye," or conjunctivitis, occurs in about 1 to 3 percent of COVID-19 cases according to the American Academy of Ophthalmology, which issued an alert advising doctors to be on the lookout for patients who complained of pink eye—with symptoms including redness, swelling, and sometimes a sticky discharge in one or both eyes—especially if they had a fever and respiratory symptoms such as cough and shortness of breath.

COVID Toes

An unusual symptom that COVID-19 patients are reporting is skin abnormalities, including purple and blue lesions on their toes, along with painful or burning sensations. Doctors have also reported a variety of measles-like skin conditions and hives-like rashes.

"Fizzing"

Some patients have reported "tingling" or "fizzing" sensations or feeling like they have a "buzzing" in the body, but these have yet to be confirmed. If they do occur, one possibility is that it may be due to an immune response.

CHAPTER 4

Getting Tested

If you are experiencing symptoms of COVID-19 or if you have been exposed to someone who is suspected or confirmed to have the illness, it is obvious you should get tested.

When the pandemic first began, getting tested for COVID-19 was difficult. But as time has progressed, this has become easier, and now there is more of a push than ever for testing.

Understanding who tests positive for coronavirus 19 can also help gauge how widely the disease has spread in a particular area and at what level the virus is still spreading, help scientists better understand the disease pattern, and also help officials monitor new outbreaks.

This chapter focuses only on diagnostic testing for COVID-19; antibody testing to determine whether people have had the virus is discussed in chapter 24.

Since the pandemic began, the Food and Drug Administration (FDA) had worked with 350 developers and authorized more than fifty tests by late April. Most of these fall into two major categories: a nose swab test and a saliva test.

Nasal Swab Test

Polymerase chain reaction tests, known as PCR, are the most common tests for determining whether someone is infected with coronavirus 19. This was the first diagnostic test, it's the most common, and it's considered the most accurate.

Every virus has a unique genetic code. For this nasal (or nasopharyngeal) swab test, a long, Q-tip-like swab is placed into one or both nostrils to collect a sample, which is then sent to a lab for testing.

There is also a throat (or oropharyngeal) swab test that requires a sample from the back of the throat.

Once the sample is collected, it can take four hours to run the test, and it could take days or weeks to receive the result.

A problem is that this test requires special supplies, expensive instruments, and highly trained technicians, so there have been logistical problems in supplying enough of them for the country.

Among other tests being developed is a quicker method using CRISPR, a genetic editing tool, that could shave the time for the original nasal swab test from five hours to forty minutes.

In a spur to increase testing, Abbott Laboratories had shipped more than one million of its "rapid" molecular tests for COVID-19 to all fifty states, which is considered a milestone in testing. The FDA granted the test "emergency use authorization" in its effort to get the test into temporary screening locations, doctor's office labs, and nursing homes. The test can deliver "positive results" in as little as five minutes and "negative results" in thirteen minutes.

The Problem of Inaccurate Test Results

Early studies of the original nasal swab test found that up to 30 percent of them reported false negatives, meaning it found people not to have COVID-19 when in fact they did.

Part of the problem is that these people may have had the disease but have been negative by the time they were tested for it. Another explanation is that the problem was caused by difficulties in collecting the samples, not the actual testing.

Accuracy has improved, but the problem has bedeviled that test and others as well.

In normal circumstances, if a test you took was negative but you were having symptoms, it would seem logical to ask to be retested. However, it is a reflection of the shortage of test kits that has led the Centers for Disease Control and Prevention (CDC) to advise that if you have symptoms but test negative, assume you have the disease and isolate yourself. But obviously, if your symptoms are getting worse, you should insist on being retested.

Saliva Test

The FDA has given emergency authorization to a saliva test for use both now at testing centers and at home with a doctor's prescription.

For this test, a person spits some saliva into a container, which is then analyzed for the virus, similar to the way DNA tests work.

Developed by a Rutgers University lab, the saliva test collects genetic material and analyzes it for the virus, just as the nasal swab test does.

In addition, the person does his or her own test, so a health care worker isn't exposed.

An early study found the saliva test to be just as accurate as the swab test, if not more so. It also uses readily available equipment, so it may not be plagued with the delays that have dogged the swab test.

Take-Home Test

With this newly authorized test, which is a variation of the nasal swab test, you receive a kit with your doctor's approval that contains a nasal swab and instructions for you to do the test at home. Proponents of these tests say that it will make testing more accessible to those who need it without possibly exposing them to others who may be ill.

Pixel by LabCorp, the first to offer at-home testing, obtained emergency authorization from the FDA to offer them first to health care workers on the front line and first responders but has plans to offer them to consumers.

There are other tests on the horizon, including an antigen test, which would look for evidence of viral genetic material, along with antibody testing to detect human antibodies against the virus. This test would both diagnose a person for COVID-19 and see if they have built up antibodies, which could help determine their immunity for the virus, so they could reenter the workforce or engage in other activities without fear of becoming infected or spreading the disease to others. (Antibody testing and the controversies surrounding it are discussed later in the book.)

But antigen tests aren't easy to make, and research to learn about the virus in order to provide the ability to make accurate tests is ongoing.

The bottom line: Even though testing capabilities have ramped up, work still needs to be done. If you need a test, contact your doctor or state health department to find out about any requirements and also which site to visit.

CHAPTER 5

How to Treat Symptoms

The pandemic has led to hospitals being overrun in some areas, like New York City, while others have plenty of capacity. Therefore, whether you are advised to stay home and treat your symptoms there or go to your local hospital's emergency department may depend on where you live.

But the following are some danger signs you shouldn't overlook, although remember to always call your doctor first before heading to the hospital.

Of course, in these times, everyone should have a thermometer on hand and check their temperature regularly.

The average normal body temperature is 98.6° Fahrenheit. When your temperature rises a few degrees above normal, it's a sign that your body is healthy and fighting infection.

The Centers for Disease Control and Prevention (CDC) hasn't developed a specific temperature pattern that can tell you whether you may have COVID-19, so in order to determine if you should be seen by a doctor or health professional, you'll be asked whether you have other symptoms associated with COVID-19 in addition to fever.

If you have a fever, call your doctor. If it's a fever of 101° Fahrenheit or lower, you will likely be told to stay home, rest, and drink plenty of fluids to avoid dehydration. But if you have a fever of 103° Fahrenheit or above, be sure to alert your doctor, as a prolonged persistent fever this high can sometimes lead to seizures or brain damage.

But should you take drugs every time you get a fever? Not necessarily. If you have a low-grade fever, you might not want to take any medication. Fever is the body's way of fighting infection, so taking medication could inhibit the body's immune response.

Instead, first try old, traditional ways to reduce the fever, such as a cool bath or lukewarm washcloths on the forehead and under the arms. And in addition, drink extra iced fluids.

But if you're very uncomfortable, you can always take a pain reliever to reduce your fever. There are two main categories of pain relievers available: acetaminophen (Tylenol and others) and a class of drugs called nonsteroidal anti-inflammatories, or NSAIDs, which includes ibuprofen (Advil, Motrin, and others), naproxen (Aleve, Anaprox, and others), indomethacin (Indocin), and aspirin.

Early research on COVID-19 out of China and France suggested that NSAIDs could make the illness worse, but the Food and Drug Administration (FDA) disagreed and says either is OK. Still, given the choice, it's probably better to play it safe and go with acetaminophen out of an abundance of caution.

Shortness of breath in COVID-19 may or may not indicate a problem. But if you are struggling to breathe or you become short of breath when lying down, call your doctor. Blue face or lips is a sign of oxygen deprivation as well.

In addition to a thermometer, you should have a pulse oximeter on hand. This is an inexpensive device that you can use on your fingertip to measure the oxygen saturation in your blood. This is to guard against possible pneumonia or pulmonary insult, which sometimes COVID-19 patients do not realize is happening until it is too late.

Most healthy people will get an oxygen reading around 95 to 98 percent. Some people with preexisting health conditions may have a lower normal reading. You should check in with your doctor if the number falls to 90 percent or lower.

If you develop symptoms of COVID-19, the CDC advises the following:
- Stay home. Most people with COVID-19 have mild illness and can recover at home without medical care. Do not leave your home, except to get medical care. Do not visit public areas.
- Take care of yourself. Get rest and stay hydrated.
- Stay in touch with your doctor. Call ahead before seeking medical care. Be sure to get care if you have trouble breathing, have any other emergency warning signs, or think it's an emergency.

- Avoid public transportation, ride-sharing, or taxis.
- Separate yourself from other people. As much as possible, stay in a specific room and away from other people and pets in your home. Also, you should use a separate bathroom, if available. If you need to be around other people or animals in or outside of the home, wear a cloth face covering.

Monitor your symptoms. Common symptoms of COVID-19 include fever and cough, as mentioned above. Difficulty breathing is a more serious symptom that means you should get medical attention.

Follow care instructions from your health care provider and local health department. Your local health authorities may give instructions on checking your symptoms and reporting information.

These are the CDC's warning signs to seek medical attention immediately:
- trouble breathing
- persistent pain or chest pressure
- new confusion or inability to rouse
- bluish lips or face

The CDC also notes that this list is not all-inclusive, and you should consult your medical provider for any symptoms that are severe or concerning to you.

The agency also says that if you have a medical emergency, you should call 911 and notify the operator that you have, or think you might have, COVID-19. If possible, cover your face until medical help arrives.

If you are at higher risk for COVID-19, ask your doctor for additional symptoms to look out for.

CHAPTER 6

Caring for Someone with COVID-19

In the case of COVID-19, people who are suspected of having the illness are told to self-quarantine for fourteen days. Also, because many cases are mild or moderate, a person may be told to quarantine at home after testing positive for the virus.

In such cases, we may find ourselves caring for someone in these circumstances. If you are taking care of someone with COVID-19, these are the recommendations the Centers for Disease Control and Prevention (CDC) says you should follow in order to care for someone who is sick:

- Help the person who is sick follow the doctor's instructions for care and medicine. For most people, symptoms last a few days, and people feel better after a week.
- See if over-the-counter medicines, such as acetaminophen, help the person feel better.
- Make sure the person who is sick drinks a lot of fluids and rests.
- Help with grocery shopping, filling prescriptions, and getting other items he or she may need. Consider having the items delivered through a delivery service, if possible.
- Take care of his or her pet(s), and limit contact between the person who is sick and the pet(s) when possible.

Often, a person with COVID-19 who has mild or moderate symptoms will recover well at home, but it is important to watch for these warning signs and always keep the doctor's phone number on hand.

These warning signs are discussed earlier, but to recap, here they are again:

- trouble breathing
- persistent pain or pressure in the chest
- new confusion or inability to rouse
- bluish lips or face

This list is not inclusive. Call the doctor if the person is getting sicker. For medical emergencies, call 911 and tell the dispatcher that the person you are calling about either might have or does have COVID-19.

You also have to take important steps to protect yourself from contracting the virus. Here are the suggestions from the Centers for Disease Control and Prevention (CDC):

- If possible, the person doing the caretaking should not be someone at higher risk for COVID-19.
- Use a separate bedroom, if possible. Have the person who is sick stay in his or her separate room, which, if possible, also has a separate bathroom.
- If you have to share a space, make sure the room has good airflow. Open a window or turn on the fan. COVID-19 spreads through respiratory droplets, and improving ventilation helps remove them from the air.
- Avoid having visitors, especially anyone who is at higher risk of COVID-19.
- Eat in separate areas. The person who is sick should eat (or be fed) in his or her room, if possible.
- Wash dishes and utensils wearing gloves and using hot water. Wash them with soap and hot water or in a dishwasher. Wash your hands thoroughly with soap and water after removing your gloves or handling used items.
- Avoid sharing personal items, including dishes, glassware, utensils, towels, bedding, or electronics.

Recommendations on When Masks and Gloves Should Be Worn

People who are sick should wear a mask (cloth face covering) when they are around at home or if they are out, such as entering a doctor's office. The covering should not be placed on young children under two, anyone who has trouble breathing, or anyone who is not able to remove the covering without help.

You, the caregiver, should wear disposable gloves when you have contact with blood, stool, or bodily fluids, such as saliva, mucus, vomit, and urine. Throw out gloves in a lined trash can.

You can wear a cloth face covering when caring for the person who is sick; however, the extent of how protective this will be is unknown as you are breathing in the virus.

Make sure you practice the other preventative actions explained elsewhere in this book: clean your hands often; avoid touching your eyes, mouth, and nose before you do; and clean and disinfect all surfaces, wearing gloves before you touch them.

Don't forget to monitor your own health for symptoms of COVID-19. If you are having trouble breathing, call 911.

CHAPTER 7

Unusual Symptoms in the Elderly

One of the most important things to know about COVID-19 is that the people who die from it tend to be at very advanced ages. It's generally assumed that this is because they have a weaker age-related immune system, but there's also a concern that these people may exhibit symptoms differently, which isn't realized until it's too late.

This is important to remember because at the beginning of the pandemic, COVID-19 ripped through senior citizen housing facilities and nursing homes, and it still shows no signs of stopping.

Fever and respiratory symptoms are considered the most common, but elderly people often exhibit these differently. They may be less sensitive to fever and exhibit lower temperatures, or a fever may be completely absent.

Respiratory symptoms may also be masked; if the person already has chronic obstructive pulmonary disease (COPD), new breathing difficulties from COVID-19 may be missed completely.

There is also anecdotal evidence that some elderly people may exhibit "atypical symptoms," some completely different than the ones ordinarily ascribed to the virus.

An article in *Kaiser Health News* explored this topic. The writer interviewed several gerontology experts, who noted that although COVID-19 is typically signaled by respiratory symptoms, including a fever, an insistent cough, and shortness of breath, older adults—the ones most at risk for complications or death from COVID-19—may display none of them.

Instead, people who are elderly may seem "off" and not act like themselves shortly after being infected by the coronavirus. They may sleep more than usual or stop eating. They may seem unusually apathetic or confused, losing orientation to their surroundings. They may become dizzy and fall. Sometimes seniors stop speaking or simply collapse.

This is how the bodies of elderly people sometimes respond to infection; their bodies may not be able to regulate temperature well, their cough reflexes may work improperly, or they may have cognitive difficulties. (Dementia is also a risk factor for COVID-19.)

Also in the elderly, their underlying chronic illnesses can mask signs of infection. For instance, a stroke survivor may have altered reflexes, or people with cognitive impairment may not be able to communicate their symptoms.

One example given in the article was of a man in his eighties who had heart disease, diabetes, and moderate cognitive impairment. Over a period of days, he stopped walking, became incontinent, and was profoundly lethargic. But he never developed a fever or a cough; his only respiratory symptom was sneezing on and off. His spouse called 911 twice, but he was checked out as OK. It was only when she insisted he be taken to the hospital that he was tested for COVID-19, and it turned out he was positive.

Recognizing these unusual signs quickly is important because if COVID-19 is the problem, the elderly may deteriorate quickly, and by the time they get help, it may be too late.

These particular symptoms have been seen in people who are elderly:

- delirium
- falls
- fatigue
- lethargy
- low blood pressure
- painful swallowing
- fainting
- diarrhea
- nausea
- vomiting
- abdominal pain
- loss of smell and taste

PART TWO

How to Prevent COVID-19

CHAPTER 8

How COVID-19 Spreads

With a disease like COVID-19, for which there is no immunity, cure, or vaccine, protecting yourself from becoming infected is the key to fighting back.

In order to understand the steps in the next section, you need to understand what we know about this disease. This will provide you with the rationale for these protection tips so that you can feel more comfortable about following them.

The major reason COVID-19 is so contagious is that people who become infected but do not show any symptoms can spread the virus for anywhere from a few days to up to two weeks! In fact, some people never develop symptoms at all but continue to spread the disease as they go about their daily lives, completely unaware.

This is much different than the flu, in which people can remain asymptomatic for only a few days before they develop symptoms, realize they are sick, and hopefully stay home and avoid spreading the disease.

These are the three ways in which COVID-19 is transmitted:

1. *Respiratory droplets transmission.* This type of transmission occurs directly, when you are coughed or sneezed on by someone who is infected. When that happens, the infected emits a small and usually wet particle cloud that stays in the air for some time. So if you are walking close by, you could inhale some of that cloud and become infected.
2. *Indirect contact transmission.* You can become infected by COVID-19 indirectly by touching a contaminated surface. For

instance, if someone walking before you should open the door by grasping the handle and you come by and touch it, the virus can transfer to your hand. If you then touch your face with that hand, the virus can enter through your eyes, nose, or mouth.

3. *Aerosol or airborne transmission.* Evidence is mounting that the coronavirus can be spread through the air. When respiratory droplets exhaled by an infected person are suspended in the air and lose water, the pathogens (infected agents) left behind form the core of the droplet, which is known as an aerosol. New evidence shows that these aerosols can fly a considerable distance—up to twenty-seven feet, one study showed. So if you come along and inhale one of these aerosols, you could be infected.

Now that you've seen how easy it is to transmit COVID-19, you can understand why these protective steps, although they seem simple, are so powerful. Remember—your number-one chance of COVID-19 infection depends on your being exposed to the virus.

The following chapters will give you the strategies you need to use to prevent being infected with coronavirus 19.

CHAPTER 9

Social Distancing

The concept of "social distancing" stems from analyzing historic data from the Spanish flu pandemic of 1918, which was the worst pandemic in modern history, and trying to determine why some municipalities suffered devastating death tolls and others, although they were not unscathed, emerged with lighter losses.

Two of the cities that are often used as examples are Minneapolis and St. Paul, which are known as the "Twin Cities."

When the first cases of Spanish flu appeared in the fall of 1918, officials in Minneapolis shut down the city on October 12, closing schools, churches, and movie theaters, and canceling large gatherings. But St. Paul remained largely open for three more weeks, its leaders believing they had the disease under control. It was only when the death toll was becoming obvious that they ordered the city shut.

Relative to the rest of the country, the two cities did not fare badly, but the death toll in Minneapolis was lighter than that in St. Paul.

Many years later, searching for ways to handle a pandemic, researchers analyzed the Spanish flu pandemic and came up with the concept of social distancing, so the Centers for Disease Control and Prevention (CDC) was ready to put this plan into action when COVID-19 struck.

Stay Home or "Shelter in Place"

Stay home or *shelter in place* are much softer terms than *lockdown*, but when we talk about staying home, not mixing with people, and avoiding crowds, these have the same historical roots as "quarantine."

The word *quarantine*, which actually means "forty days," is a state of isolation that is imposed to keep a disease from spreading. When

COVID-19 broke out in China, the government took forcible steps to isolate Wuhan, the city where the disease was first identified. This was referred to as a "lockdown."

In the United States, this concept has been softened, and for the most part, people have been instructed mostly to keep to themselves. These efforts have been paying off, with case numbers and death rates declining in some of the areas, like New York City, that were hit hardest by COVID-19.

Social Distancing

Social distancing, or physical distancing, is a set of measures used to prevent the spread of a contagious disease by maintaining a physical space between people.

Whenever people are out in public, the CDC advocates that they keep to this social distance or physical distance of six feet between themselves and others.

This makes sense because that was believed how far the respiratory droplets travel when someone infected with COVID-19 coughs or sneezes.

Researchers now believe that COVID-19 can travel much farther than that, so should you increase your distance?

Dr. Donald Milton, a professor of environmental health at the University of Maryland's school of public health, said in an interview with the American Chemical Society on COVID-19 that there's no "magic number," but generally six feet seems like a reasonable distance to stand, especially if both people are wearing masks, which are discussed in chapter 11.

However, if you are at higher risk of COVID-19 complications, and especially if the virus is spreading in your community, you may want to adjust your distance accordingly, possibly to twelve feet.

Another good way to complement social distancing is to cut down on nonessential errands or daily trips. However, as these regulations ease, you will have to decide how much risk you want to take in going out and about.

Social Distancing and Pets

When the pandemic began, amusing images of cats and dogs wearing surgical masks popped up on the internet, but it turns out that the subject of COVID-19 and animals is no joke.

The CDC still says that COVID-19 is spread primarily from person to person, but the agency is now recommending that pet owners observe the same type of social distancing guideline they do for themselves with their animals.

The agency listed the new guidelines after a few, very rare cases in which dogs and cats became infected with the virus from their owners.

The guidelines call for owners to restrict their pets from interacting with other animals when outside their homes and urge people to keep cats indoors when possible and to walk dogs on a leash while maintaining a distance of six feet from other people and animals.

The agency also calls for pet owners to avoid dog parks or public places where a large number of people and dogs gather.

The CDC stressed that in the United States, there is no evidence that animals are playing "a significant role" in the spread of the disease.

CHAPTER 10

Handwashing

It may seem like a simple practice, but thoroughly washing your hands frequently throughout the day is a surprisingly effective way of preventing COVID-19.

Sure, there was a run on hand sanitizer at the start of the pandemic, and stores were sold out. But don't worry; although sanitizer is convenient, when it comes to the handwashing that prevents COVID-19, soap is your better bet.

The coronavirus is a pathogen that is coated in a fatty lipid covering, which soap can penetrate and break up, especially when combined with the rubbing action of your hands. In fact, it's the rubbing you do that really makes handwashing effective, because this action actually breaks up the virus on a molecular level.

Here's the Centers for Disease Control and Prevention (CDC) method for handwashing. Wet your hands with clean running water and apply soap. Rub your hands together to lather them, and then scrub all the surfaces of your hands, including the palms, backs, fingers, between the fingers, and under the nails. Keep scrubbing for at least twenty seconds, and as you've no doubt heard, you can time yourself by singing the "Happy Birthday" song twice. Then dry your hands using a clean towel or a paper towel or air dry them.

Now, if you're using hand sanitizer, the CDC has this important advice as well. Use an alcohol-based hand sanitizer that contains at least 60 percent alcohol. Put enough of the product on your hands to cover all the surfaces. Rub your hands together until they feel dry, which should take about the same twenty seconds. Don't rinse or wipe off the hand sanitizer until it's dry, because it may not work as well.

Handwashing is also an important part of good personal hygiene. If you cough or sneeze, cover your mouth or nose with a tissue or towel and avoid touching your eyes, nose, or mouth afterward, and then thoroughly wash your hands with soap and water.

The CDC suggests these additional key times for washing your hands:

- after blowing your nose, coughing, or sneezing
- after using the bathroom
- before eating or preparing food
- before and after contact with pets
- before and after providing care for another person (e.g., a child)

CHAPTER 11

When to Wear a Mask

During the COVID-19 pandemic, no topic has raised more confusion than that of masks.

At the start of the pandemic, the Centers for Disease Control and Prevention (CDC) specifically stated the public had no need to wear masks and indeed should not. Then, after it became apparent that the virus was more contagious than originally thought, the agency did a turnabout and declared masks should be worn.

But they stuck to their contention that the type that people should wear are cloth masks, which can be purchased or homemade, and to underscore the difference between this and a medical-grade mask, they called it a "face covering."

This is because medical-grade and surgical masks are in short supply and are needed for first responders, like EMTs, doctors, and nurses, who work with people who are infected.

Here is a rundown on how different types of masks stack up in terms of offering protection against COVID-19.

N95 masks. Also known as respirators, these masks come in two types: with or without breathing tubes. This type of mask is the most effective against the coronavirus. The masks with breathing tubes are more comfortable for people with chronic respiratory diseases, heart disease, or other ailments that make breathing more difficult. The masks with breathing tubes, however, shouldn't be worn by people who actually work in contact with people infected with COVID-19.

Surgical masks. These are basic protective gear for health care professionals and medical personnel. These single-use masks will protect you from actual droplets if you are coughed or sneezed on. These have been in short supply during the pandemic, and again, consumers are urged not to purchase them because they are needed by health care workers. But unlike respirators, they can sometimes be available for purchase.

Cloth masks. These are the masks the CDC recommends that people in general should use during the pandemic. They can be purchased commercially, or you can make them at home.

The problem, though, is that cloth masks are not that effective—they can allow for as much as 97 percent of viral particles to enter, which means virtually no protection for the wearer at all. In fact, these masks are better at protecting others who come into contact with you, not the other way around. So while most are better than nothing, they can give you a false sense of security.

Should N95 masks become available and you have the opportunity to get one without depriving a health care worker, go for it, as COVID-19 is apt to be with us for a long time. But even should N95 masks remain unavailable, surgical masks are becoming less scarce, so if you have the opportunity to buy some, do so, as they are more effective than cloth masks.

As for cloth masks, there are some ways to make them more effective at protecting you from the coronavirus.

How to Make a Better Mask

Homemade masks can play a role in the fight against COVID-19, but much depends on the material they are made from, so researchers at Wake Forest Baptist Health set out to find the best ones.

Their goal was to find out which type of mask best removed particles 0.3 to 1.0 microns in diameter, the size of many viruses and bacteria, in comparison to standard surgical masks and N95 respirator masks.

They found that the effectiveness of homemade masks varied widely; the best achieved 79 percent filtration as compared to surgical masks (62 percent to 65 percent) and N95 masks (97 percent). But other homemade masks tested performed significantly worse, sometimes demonstrating as little as 1 percent filtration.

To make the most effective mask, use two layers of "quilter's cotton," with a thread count of 180 or more, and material with an especially tight weave, like batik. A double-layer mask with a simple cotton outer layer and an inner layer of flannel also performed well, they said. These materials are better than simple cotton, or even doubling that up, they say.

They also suggest holding the fabric up to the light; if you can see through it, the material is not tightly woven enough.

Remember, don't let wearing a mask give you a false sense of security. Always wash your hands often and observe social distancing.

How to Put on Your Mask

Making sure your mask fits well and does not become contaminated when you put it on and take it off is very important.

Wash your hands before putting it on. Make sure the mask fits closely enough to go over your nose and mouth with no gaps. Then place the ear loops around your ears. When you are ready to remove your mask, wash your hands thoroughly before doing so. Push the front side of the mask with one hand while holding the ear loops, and remove them from each ear separately. Then wash your hands thoroughly again.

Special Considerations

If you are pregnant, elderly, or have a chronic health condition that makes it difficult for you to breathe, ask your doctor if you should wear a mask or face covering.

Regarding children, it was first thought that they couldn't become infected by the coronavirus, but we know that is not true. While most children may not get very sick, if they are infected, they can still transmit the disease. If you want them to wear a mask during times of heavy spread, make sure you select one that is specially made for their smaller faces.

CHAPTER 12

When to Wear Gloves

Second only to questions about masks is the confusion over whether or not to wear disposable gloves. During the pandemic, they were, like medical masks, in short supply.

The Centers for Disease Control and Prevention (CDC) says gloves are not necessary and should be worn only if you are in danger of being directly in contact with the virus, such as if you're caring for someone with COVID-19.

Here are some instances where wearing gloves makes sense:

- when in the grocery store, handling items that have been touched by others
- pumping gas at the gas station
- when cleaning and disinfecting your home
- if caring for someone who is a suspected or confirmed COVID-19 patient

But if you are going to wear disposable gloves, it's important that you know how to wear them and dispose of them properly; otherwise, you may just end up contaminating yourself.

Here are tips for when you are wearing gloves:

- Make sure your gloves fit properly. Too-tight gloves will break, and too-loose gloves won't protect you well enough.
- Change them often. You need to change your gloves every time you wash or sanitize your hands; otherwise, you risk contamination.

- Remove them safely. Use one gloved hand to carefully peel off the other, and then use the forefinger of the bare hand to slide the second glove off, wedging the finger inside the wrist of the gloves and never touching the outside surface.
- Never sanitize the gloves; doing that only transfers germs on the gloves to your sanitizer container.
- Safely dispose of gloves in a trash container or put them in a bag until you can reach a trash bag.
- Wash your hands thoroughly after removing and disposing of the gloves.
- Don't reuse gloves; their effectiveness wanes the more you use them.
- Don't let wearing gloves give you a false sense of security.
- Still observe social distancing and wear a mask to avoid touching your face.

There is also a controversy over whether disposable gloves should be worn by grocery store clerks. Some say yes, but others argue they can lead to cross-contamination from handling many items in the store.

According to the CDC, grocery store employees should wear cloth masks, but gloves are not necessary if proper handwashing and/or sanitizing procedures are employed.

CHAPTER 13

Food Shopping, Takeout, and Delivery

If you are in an area that is still having outbreaks, and especially if you're at risk, you may want to forego a trip to the grocery store and have your groceries delivered.

But generally, going to these stores is safe as long as you take these precautions:

- Make a list ahead of time of all the items you need so you can be in and out of the store quickly.
- Wear your mask always.
- Wear gloves and trash them when you get home.
- Take advantage of special hours for senior citizens and people at risk.
- Look around the store and make sure they are taking precautions as well. This includes having employees wear masks, sanitizing carts, taking care to make sure the aisles are not crowded, and enforcing social distancing at checkout counters. If this is not the case, this isn't where you should be doing your shopping.
- Wash your hands thoroughly with soap and water when you get home.
- Don't touch your face when you are out in public.

What about Takeout Meals?

For many people, during the pandemic, getting takeout meals from their favorite eateries proved to be an enjoyable way of dealing with some of the restrictions and also supporting these businesses.

But what precautions should you take? Although people tend to worry about the virus spreading in their food, that doesn't happen because there is no evidence that food produced in the United States can transmit coronavirus 19, the Food and Drug Administration (FDA) says.

But you can get infected if you touch something that has been contaminated by a restaurant worker or delivery person who has COVID-19 and then take it to your house. This is why many eateries have refined "contactless delivery" systems and will deliver food to your door, which is preferable to you picking it up in person.

Rather than worry about the food itself, focus on the outside packaging, because it is here where the virus may be lurking.

Here are tips that Olga Padilla-Zakour, director of the Cornell Food Venture Center at Cornell University, shared with National Public Radio:

- Create a safe food environment in your home to place your food when it arrives by cleaning any surfaces it may touch.
- Pay (and tip) in advance by phone to minimize person-to-person interaction when the food arrives.
- Let the delivery person leave the food at your doorstep. Wait until the delivery person is at least six feet away before retrieving the food.
- Remove the food from the takeout bags or containers and dispose of or recycle them appropriately.
- After disposing of packaging, wash your hands for twenty seconds with soap and water.
- Wipe counters and other surfaces where you unpacked the food.

CHAPTER 14

Disinfecting Your Home

Because you can contract coronavirus indirectly by touching an item contaminated with the virus, disinfecting your home is very important during an outbreak and is also good practice generally.

A study published recently in the medical journal *Lancet* showed that the virus can remain on some objects for up to seven days. Here are their findings:

- printed and tissue paper—three hours
- cardboard—one day
- wood—two days
- cloth fabric—two days
- paper money or glass—four days
- stainless steel, plastic, and (surprisingly) surgical masks—seven days

Cleaning removes dirt and germs, but in order to eliminate the virus, you need to disinfect. According to the article, these ingredients will kill the coronavirus within five minutes:

- household bleach
- 70 percent ethanol (rubbing alcohol)
- 7.5 percent povidone-iodine
- 0.05 percent chloroxylenol
- 0.05 percent chlorhexidine
- 0.1 percent benzalkonium chloride

Many antiseptic solutions and detergents contain one or more of these ingredients. The exact concentrations of each ingredient vary from product to product, so label reading is important.

It's also important to remember that these chemicals are strong, so don't poison yourself while doing this! Calls to state and local poison control centers rose 20 percent during the first month of the pandemic, the Centers for Disease Control and Prevention (CDC) reports. To avoid harmful exposure, the agency recommends that users remember these cautions:

- Follow label directions.
- Don't mix chemicals.
- Wear skin and eye protection.
- Use in a well-ventilated area.
- Store chemicals out of the reach of children.

Shoes

Studies have shown that you can pick up the virus on your shoes and then bring it into your house. A simple way to avoid this is to pick a pair of shoes to wear outdoors and then remove them before entering your home and leave them outside—in a garage, for example. If you need to take them inside, you can, while wearing gloves, wipe them down with disinfectant or store them in a sealed plastic bag. Be sure to wash your hands thoroughly afterward and avoid touching your face until you do.

Smartphone

Most of us are never without our mobile phones—outside included— so they can potentially become one of the most contaminated items we touch. Both Apple and Samsung warn against using harsh cleaners on their products.

According to an article on CNET, Apple says you can use a 70 percent isopropyl alcohol wipe or Clorox Disinfecting Wipe on the surface of any of their products, but don't use bleach, avoid getting moisture into any port or opening, and don't submerge the item in any cleaning agents.

Regarding Samsung products, the company also warns against using bleach but says you can also use a disinfectant, such as a hypochlorous acid–based solution (containing 50–80 ppm) or an alcohol-based solution (containing more than 70 percent ethanol or isopropyl alcohol). Do not apply these liquid solutions directly to your device; they should be carefully applied to a microfiber cloth instead.

Laundry

In these days of COVID-19, the most mundane tasks have become challenging. In most cases, unless you are caring for or in contact with someone infected, your clothes shouldn't be a main concern.

But as a regular hygienic practice, changing out of clothing you've worn outside is a good idea. This is especially true if you are using public transportation or you are working outside.

Here are the CDC's recommendations.

For clothing, towels, linens, and other items:

- Launder items according to the manufacturer's instructions. Use the warmest appropriate water setting and dry items completely.
- Wear disposable gloves when handling dirty laundry from a person who is sick.
- Dirty laundry from a person who is sick can be washed with other people's items.
- Do not shake dirty laundry.
- Clean and disinfect clothes hampers.
- When you're done, remove your gloves, dispose of them, and immediately wash your hands thoroughly.

CHAPTER 15

Traveling Safely

The pandemic highlighted the risks of air travel and cruise ships. Global air travel was blamed for spreading the virus throughout the world, and borders were shut down. Horrifying stories of passengers getting sick on cruise ships filled the news.

But the economic crisis caused by the pandemic has also driven travel prices down, so now everyone is wondering when it will be safe to travel again.

No matter whether or not a pandemic is occurring, travel raises the risk of getting sick. So if you are planning a trip and you're at risk for COVID-19, or even the seasonal flu, you should consult your doctor first.

An analysis of twenty-seven studies published a few years ago in the *Journal of Travel Medicine* looked at airplanes, cruise ships, trains, and busses as modes of increased transmission of the flu, severe acute respiratory syndrome (SARS), and Middle East respiratory syndrome (MERS) and found various evidence of all of these as the means of transmitting disease.

So if you're thinking of traveling, check the Centers for Disease Control and Prevention (CDC) Coronavirus 2019 Information for Travel website (https://www.cdc.gov/coronavirus/2019-ncov/travelers/index.html), which rates the risk per country on an interactive world map. The site also lists which countries have travel alerts and ranks them according to seriousness.

It turns out that your main danger is not so much from the recycled air, as that is efficiently filtered, but from being in close proximity to fellow passengers who may be infected.

Also, there are various surfaces on planes, including the airplane tray, seat buckles, and magazine pockets, that could become contaminated.

If you are at high risk for COVID-19, you should steer clear of flying whenever the disease is spreading. If you do choose to fly, observe all the precautions you would ordinarily—limit what you touch, wear a mask, bring along hand sanitizer, and try not to touch your face.

When it comes to cruises, that industry realizes it will have to do a lot to erase the memory of the horrific headlines that accompanied the pandemic. In this case, a lot will depend on what restrictions the cruise industry takes to convince prospective passengers that it is safe to go back on their boats. But your job is to not be seduced by the bargain rates they will no doubt offer unless you are certain that COVID-19 is no longer spreading—anywhere! Remember, cruise passengers are likely to come from anywhere in the world.

But what about just getting around town? Some people don't have the option of a car and, even in times of disease outbreak, may simply need to get around. What measure of safety are you giving up if you travel by Uber, Lyft, a rental car, or a cab?

Consumer Reports looked at those options and came up with suggestions. Even though car-sharing services are investing in heavy-duty cleaning equipment, a taxi may be your best bet if it has a partition between you and the driver.

If you're planning to travel by car, AARP has some excellent tips. Make sure you clean and sanitize your car, and take cleaning supplies, disposable gloves, tissues, and your mask along. As noted before, wear disposable gloves when pumping gas, and use your credit card at the pump to avoid person-to-person interaction. You can always disinfect the card afterward.

If you need to use a public bathroom, be careful not to touch fixtures like the faucet or door handle after thoroughly washing your hands, and since these restrooms often don't have soap, make sure you've brought it (or some hand sanitizer) along.

During the pandemic, domestic travel was discouraged, but staying at a hotel or inn is now becoming feasible. But for stays longer than one night, contact the front desk and ask to forgo housekeeping services, allowing you to do your own sanitation and limit the number of people going in and out of your room during your stay, AARP suggests.

For shorter trips, Uber, Lyft, and other ride-sharing services have also discontinued rides shared between passengers who don't know each other, but whether or not this service is offered, you are better off riding solo.

Whether you're in your own car, a ride share, or a taxi, crack open the window for better ventilation, even if everyone is feeling fine.

PART THREE

Get Healthy to Fight COVID-19

CHAPTER 16

Sleep Is the Key to Immunity

No matter what your age, you need eight to ten hours of sleep a night.

Ironically, it seems that the more sleep we need, the less we get, but if you don't get all the sleep you need, both in quantity and in quality, then you are putting your health—and your immunity—at risk.

According to the Centers for Disease Control and Prevention (CDC), an estimated fifty to seventy million Americans do not get enough sleep.

Sleep not only plays a key factor in traffic and industrial accidents; it also increases the risk of high blood pressure, diabetes, obesity, and cardiovascular disease, which are all risk factors for severe COVID-19 complications as well.

But worst of all, research shows that not getting enough sleep also damages your immune system!

While no studies yet exist on the relationship between sleep and COVID-19, several studies done over the years show that not enough sleep translates to a higher vulnerability to the flu.

For instance, one study, done a few years ago and published in the journal *Behavioral Sleep Medicine*, found that healthy college students who suffered from various sleep problems, including insomnia, mounted a weaker response to the flu vaccine. This translated into a higher risk of them catching the flu and getting sicker, the researchers said.

And the Mayo Clinic recently reported, "Studies show that people who don't get quality sleep or enough sleep are more likely to get sick after being exposed to a virus, such as a common cold virus. Lack of sleep can also affect how fast you recover if you do get sick. During sleep, your immune system releases proteins called cytokines, some of which help promote sleep. Certain cytokines need to increase when you have an infection or inflammation, or when you're under stress. Sleep deprivation may decrease production of these protective cytokines. In addition, infection-fighting antibodies and cells are reduced during periods when you don't get enough sleep."

Obstructive Sleep Apnea and COVID-19

One of the conditions that can rob you of sound sleep is obstructive sleep apnea, or simply "sleep apnea," which is a common sleep disorder.

There is no evidence at this time that having sleep apnea raises your risk of COVID-19, according to Dr. Rajkumar (Raj) Desgupta, M.D., F.A.C.P., a certified sleep specialist.

Most people who have sleep apnea are overweight, however, so losing weight will not only lower your risk of COVID-19 but also help you sleep better.

If you have been diagnosed with moderate to severe sleep apnea, it's very likely that you use a CPAP machine to manage your condition. A CPAP machine is a kind of oxygen mask that delivers air through the nose at a high enough pressure to keep the airways open.

Because there has been a focus on ventilators since the start of the COVID-19 pandemic, a lot of people who use CPAP machines have become confused and are wondering if they should stop, says Dr. Desgupta. However, if you've been prescribed a CPAP machine, it is important for you to keep using it and keeping it clean, he says.

"In order to get enough sleep, you need the right quantity of sleep and the right quality of sleep. And if you're not using your CPAP because you have obstructive sleep apnea, you're going to further weaken your immune system," he adds.

How to Get a Good Night's Sleep

Of course, anxiety about your health, like that evoked by COVID-19, can translate into difficulty sleeping. Here are some suggestions on how to get a good night's sleep no matter the circumstances:

- Get enough sleep. Determine the duration of sleep you need and prioritize that each night.

- Go to sleep and wake up at the same time daily. Your body craves predictability and order.
- Try not to nap.
- Create a comfortable environment. Make sure your bedroom is separate from your workspace and conducive to sleep. Darken the room, keep the temperature cool, use an eye mask, and try a white noise machine to block noise or distractions.
- Turn off your smartphone two hours before bedtime, don't recharge it near your bed, and don't read a book on an electronic device—the blue light has been found to disturb sleep cycles.
- If sleep is a problem, don't drink coffee or tea, eat chocolate, or use any stimulants past noon.
- Avoid alcohol at night; even if you think it relaxes you, drinking alcohol actually increases your chance of awakening during the night.
- Try melatonin as a sleep aid. Start with the lowest dosage you can find.

CHAPTER 17

What to Eat for a Better Immune System

To fight back against COVID-19, you need a strong immune system. Your immune system is complicated. It's not a single organ; it's a complex network of cells and proteins that act together to defend your body against infection.

There isn't a single step you can take to improve your immune system, but there are several different actions you can take to help strengthen and better balance it in order to help it guard against viral onslaught, such as coronavirus 19.

By now, you've learned how contagious COVID-19 is and how strategies you implement can put you out of harm's way from this infection.

Now it's time to learn how to make your body stronger so that you can better withstand the assault of COVID-19 should you become infected.

This chapter on nutrition, along with those on sleep (chapter 16), exercise (chapter 19), and stress (chapter 20), can all, acting together, help bolster and better balance your immune system.

When it comes to eating, "Dr. Crandall's Life Plan Diet"—the culmination of Dr. Crandall's four decades of practice in cardiology, along with his experience traveling the world and learning the ancient secrets of people in Africa, Asia, and elsewhere around the globe— is an excellent way to eat, whether you want to lose weight, build up your immune system, or simply cut through all the nonsense surrounding food and find a good, clean way to eat. The diet is outlined in Dr. Crandall's book *The Simple Heart Cure* (Humanix Books, updated edition, 2019).

These are the principles you can use to build your meals for a day of healthy eating.

First, fill up on fruits and vegetables because they are packed with vitamins and minerals, including antioxidants, that will not only help satisfy your appetite but also keep your immune system strong. Even during times of viral spread, when you want to stay indoors and shopping or online ordering options are limited, your goal should always be to buy fresh fruits and vegetables that have been grown organically and without pesticides.

When you are dressing a salad, use high-quality olive oil. Olive oil is a monounsaturated fat, meaning it's a "good" fat and is rich in antioxidants and also polyphenols that have been shown to have antiviral activities.

Make sure to eat enough protein. Although this diet is largely plant-based, there is some animal-based protein, particularly fish. Fish that are rich in omega-3 oils, like wild salmon or rainbow trout, are an excellent source of protein, for example. Goat cheese and nonfat hard cheeses, as well as an occasional egg, can provide protein also. As for red meat, limit it to special occasions. Preferably wild game or venison are also good choices.

The best way to supercharge your immune system is to choose foods already imbued by nature with illness-fighting powers. The foods you eat interact with your immune system through your microbiome, the trillions of microbes that reside in our gut and interact with each other in a mutually beneficial way.

These delicious foods help boost the immune system:

- *Red bell peppers.* Peppers are very high in vitamin C, and just one provides 170 percent of the daily recommended allowance. Yellow and red peppers have more antioxidants than green ones.
- *Sunflower seeds.* Sunflower seeds are high in vitamin E.
- *Broccoli.* Broccoli is an excellent source of vitamin C, along with antioxidants and phytochemicals that support the immune system.

- *Mushrooms.* These delicious fungi are one of the few dietary sources of vitamin D, and a study on eating shiitake mushrooms shows they improve immunity better than any pharmaceutical drug on the market.
- *Yogurt.* Yogurt is a great source of probiotics, which are a source of good bacteria to promote a healthy gut and immune system.
- *Spinach.* Spinach is rich in vitamin C and antioxidants and has beta-carotene, which also supports healthy immune system functioning.
- *Strawberries.* Strawberries are another vitamin C powerhouse.

Eliminate These Immunity Killers

The other part of your strategy to keep your immunity system strong is to make certain that everything you do is designed to enhance your body's immunity response. Therefore, you need to root out the foods you eat or the behaviors you engage in that can weaken your immune system.

Refined Sugar

As you've seen, obesity is one of the biggest risk factors in developing serious complications, and even dying, from COVID-19. People who eat a lot of refined sugar, in cakes, candy, pies, and the like, are far more likely to become obese, and obesity produces inflammation, which damages the immune system.

But when it comes to COVID-19, there is an even more worrisome effect. While there have not been studies on obesity and COVID-19 directly, research published on the swine flu pandemic of 2009 looked at this issue because obesity raised the risk of severe complications in this viral disease as well.

People who contracted the swine flu were also at a major increased risk for severe complications and death if they were obese. A study published in the *Journal of Infectious Diseases* the year following that pandemic explored that issue and found that obesity created several problems, but one of the most dangerous was that it raised the probability of a cytokine storm. This is the overreaction of the immune system that occurs late in the course of COVID-19 and can lead to death. One of the easiest ways to avoid obesity is to eliminate sugar from your diet.

Smoking

During the pandemic, many people turned to smoking as a way to deal with their anxiety and to calm themselves, whether it was by smoking tobacco products, e-cigarettes, or marijuana.

But if you chose to do this, it's time to kick the habit. Because the coronavirus attacks the lungs, it makes sense that you would want them to be as healthy as possible.

A recent study in the *New England Journal of Medicine* looked at coronavirus patients in China and found that those who smoked were twice as likely than nonsmokers to have severe lung infections. One possible reason for this is that smoking increases the amount of ACE2 receptors in the lungs, and that is the cell site that the virus attacks.

As for vaping, there has been concern over the use of e-cigarettes, especially since last summer, when it was linked to a lung disease that sickened numerous users, especially those who were young.

Reports also say that marijuana use rose during the pandemic, especially in municipalities where smoke shops are considered "essential."

But according to Dr. Albert Rizzo, a pulmonologist and chief medical officer for the American Lung Association, smoking cannabis inflames the airways similar to the way bronchitis does.

The bottom line is, when it comes to your lungs, whether you choose tobacco, e-cigarettes, or marijuana, you won't be doing your lungs any good, and there is also evidence they dampen the immune system.

Alcoholic Beverages

Alcoholic beverage use soared during the pandemic, with beverage sales rising by 55 percent by the third week of March—ample evidence that people were either turning to or stockpiling booze to see themselves through.

But if you want to marshal all your defenses against the coronavirus, turning to liquor is not a wise thing to do.

Too much alcohol can worsen high blood pressure, cause heartbeat irregularities, raise blood sugar levels in people with diabetes, and also overstress the liver, all conditions that have been demonstrated to raise the risk of COVID-19 complications.

In addition, clinicians have long observed an association between excessive alcohol consumption and immune-related health effects, such as the susceptibility to pneumonia, and in recent years, such abuse has been linked to acute respiratory distress syndrome (ARDS), sepsis, alcoholic liver disease, and slower or incomplete recovery from infection, as well as other ailments.

Since you need your immune system operating at peak capabilities to ward off potential COVID-19 infection, it's obvious that overindulging in alcohol is not the way to go, in times of pandemic or not.

CHAPTER 18

Supplements to Boost Immunity

Overnight, the pandemic changed the way we eat and choose our foods.

We were told to limit our trips to the supermarket, farmer's markets were shut down, and people became more focused on buying bathroom tissue and hand sanitizer than fresh fruits and vegetables. But even under the best of circumstances, the nutritional content of our food has deteriorated over the decades. Nowadays, agriculture is known as "agribusiness," and the accent is on business. Technology speeds the growing cycle but leaches the nutrients from the soil.

To fight back against COVID-19, you need every weapon you can lay your hands on, and this means taking supplements, which can give you an important nutritional edge. These recommendations can strengthen your immune system to help fight off COVID-19.

These are the essential supplements you need to keep your immune system strong. They are also useful if you feel the symptoms of a cold, the flu, or even what you suspect might be COVID-19 coming on.

It's also always important to take a multivitamin every day to cover any deficiencies you might have of which you are unaware.

Vitamin C

Vitamin C is the go-to vitamin to help protect against infection due to its important role in immune health. It is also necessary for cellular death, which helps keep your immune system healthy by clearing out old cells and replacing them with new ones, and it functions as a powerful antioxidant, protecting against damage caused by oxidative stress that occurs with aging.

Several studies have found that vitamin C, taken before and during respiratory illnesses, may help ease symptoms and shorten duration.

A large study, published in the *Cochrane Database System Review*, found that regularly supplementing with vitamin C at an average dose reduced the duration of colds by 8 percent in adults and 14 percent in children.

Intravenous vitamin C is also being used against COVID-19 and has been found to significantly improve the health of people with severe infections, including sepsis and acute respiratory distress syndrome (ARDS), which are two of the deadliest complications that can occur in COVID-19.

Foods high in vitamin C: broccoli, cantaloupe, cauliflower, kale, kiwi, papaya, sweet potato, strawberries, tomato, and citrus fruits, including oranges, mandarins, and limes.

Take: 500 to 1,000 mg of vitamin C daily.

✓ Vitamin D3

Vitamin D3 is a nutrient essential to the health and functioning of the immune system. Vitamin D3 enhances the pathogen-fighting effects of your body's white blood cells, which decrease inflammation and help promote the immune response. Deficiency in vitamin D3 is linked to COVID-19.

But many people are deficient in this vitamin. It is known as the "sunshine vitamin," but as we age, our ability to synthesize vitamin D3 through our skin from the sun diminishes, so many older people are found to be deficient, even if they live in sunny climates like Florida.

In a 2019 review of randomized controlled studies in more than eleven thousand people, as reported in the *Health Technology Assessment Journal*, vitamin D3 supplementation significantly decreased respiratory infections in people who were deficient in this vitamin and lowered infection risk in those with adequate vitamin D3 levels.

Foods high in vitamin D3: salmon, herring and sardines, tuna (fresh or canned), egg yolks (preferably organic or free-range), and mushrooms.

Take: 5,000 IU of vitamin D3 daily for three months, and then get a vitamin D3 level check at the end of three months to readjust the dosage.

✓ Vitamin A

Vitamin A is the generic term for a group of fat-soluble compounds that are highly important for human health and essential to many processes in the body, including maintaining a balanced immune system. Among its many functions is aiding in the production and functioning of white blood cells, which clear bacteria and other pathogens from your bloodstream. This means a deficiency in vitamin A can increase your susceptibility to infection and delay your recovery when you get sick. A study in the *Annual Review of Nutrition* found that in countries where infections like measles and malaria are common, correcting vitamin A deficiencies in children was shown to decrease their risk of dying from these diseases.

Foods high in vitamin A: broccoli, black-eyed peas, red peppers, spinach, sweet potatoes, mango, cantaloupe, tomato juice, dried apricots, and pumpkin.

Take: 25,000 IU of vitamin A daily.

Zinc

Zinc is a vital mineral that is commonly made into lozenges meant to boost your immune system. This helps the immune system fight off invading bacteria and viruses.

Most colds are caused by a type of virus called rhinovirus, which thrives and multiplies in the nasal passages and throat (upper respiratory system). Zinc may work by preventing the rhinovirus from multiplying. It may also stop the rhinovirus from lodging in the mucous membranes of the throat and nose.

A zinc deficiency affects your immune system's ability to function properly, resulting in an increased risk of infection and disease, including pneumonia in the elderly, according to a study published in *Nutrition Reviews*.

Food high in zinc: Lean meats (preferably grass-fed), shellfish (oysters, Alaskan crab, shrimp, mussels), legumes, seeds, nuts, eggs, whole grains, and dairy foods, especially milk and cheese.

Take: Up to 40 mg a day. If you feel symptoms coming on, you can take one lozenge containing 18.75 mg of zinc acetate up to four times a day.

✓Garlic

Garlic has been used for centuries as both a flavoring for food and a medicine. Garlic offers many health benefits, including a lowered risk of heart disease and improved mental health, and most importantly, it helps the immune system ward off the common cold and flu.

Garlic contains a compound called alliin, which, when crushed or chewed, turns into allicin, the main active ingredient in garlic.

A study at the University of Edinburgh looked at a chemical in garlic that is believed to kill bacteria that cause life-threatening lung infections in people with cystic fibrosis. Current therapies available to treat these infections, which are potentially fatal, are limited and require the use of combinations of three or four antibiotics at a time.

The researchers found that allicin inhibited the growth of the disease-causing bacteria by modifying key enzymes, which deactivated them and halted important biological processes within their cells.

Take: 9,000 to 18,000 mg of high-allicin garlic supplements or add a clove of garlic to a recipe that you are making daily.

✓ Selenium

This is a trace element that is essential for health and plays more than two dozen roles in the human body, including for reproduction and thyroid hormone metabolism. Selenium is an antioxidant, and it also is anti-inflammatory and antiviral. Selenium has also been reported to slow immune dysfunction. You also especially need selenium if you have HIV or are undergoing kidney dialysis.

In a study published in the *Archives of Internal Medicine*, researchers reported the results of their research, which found that a daily selenium supplement is associated with suppression of the progression of HIV viral load and improvement of immune function in patients infected with human immunodeficiency virus 1 (HIV-1).

Foods high in selenium: Brazil nuts, fish, turkey, chicken, cottage cheese, eggs, brown rice, sunflower seeds, mushrooms, oatmeal, spinach, lentils, cashews, bananas, milk, and yogurt.

Take: 200 mcg of selenium daily.

Probiotics

Probiotics are beneficial microorganisms that live in your gut, and by adding healthy ones, you can balance out negative ones and achieve certain health benefits, including to the immune system. There is emerging evidence that *Bifidobacterium* and *Lactobacillus* can boost the immune system's response to viral illness.

One study of *Bifidobacterium* found that in older people, it reduced the influence of influenza and fever in an at-risk population compared with study participants who received a placebo, according to research published in the journal *Bioscience Biotechnology*. Also, a study on *Lactobacillus* published in *Frontiers in Pharmacology* found it helped reduce the duration of respiratory infections.

Foods that contain probiotics: yogurt, kefir, kombucha, sauerkraut, pickles, miso, tempeh, kimchi, and sourdough bread.

Take: A probiotic brand that has a higher number of probiotics (high-CFU count), ideally at least fifty billion per serving. Also select a probiotic supplement that has ten or more probiotic strains, such as *Bacillus coagulans*, *Lactobacillus acidophilus*, *Bifidobacterium*, and *Streptococcus thermophilus* strains.

Magnesium

The fourth most abundant mineral in the body, magnesium is involved in literally hundreds of biochemical reactions in your body; in fact, every one of your cells needs magnesium to function properly. It benefits people with diabetes, high blood pressure, and heartbeat irregularities (all underlying COVID-19 risk factors), and it's also anti-inflammatory.

People with diabetes are at risk for serious complications, and death, from COVID-19. A review by researchers at Northwestern University, published in the journal *Circulation*, suggested that magnesium addresses several components of metabolic syndrome, a collection of conditions that includes obesity and diabetes, by favorably impacting blood glucose levels and insulin action.

Foods high in magnesium: dark chocolate (70 percent cocoa or higher), avocados, nuts, legumes, tofu, seeds, whole grains, and fatty fish (salmon, mackerel, halibut).

Take: 200 to 400 mg of magnesium daily.

Quercetin

This is a flavonoid, which means it is one of a diverse group of phytonutrients (plant chemicals) found in almost all fruits and vegetables. Along with carotenoids, they are responsible for the vivid colors in fruits and vegetables. Flavonoids are the largest group of phytonutrients, with more than six thousand types.

Quercetin is known for its antiaging, life-extending benefits, and it also prevents DNA damage and supports the natural stress response, but it really excels as an immunity booster and infection fighter.

Quercetin kills viruses in laboratory dish experiments, and it has in-hibited hepatitis C virus replication. Also, in one study, reported in *Antiviral Research Journal*, quercetin blocked replication of the rhino-virus, the virus responsible for the common cold.

Foods high in quercetin: onions, apples, grapes, broccoli, citrus fruits, cherries, tea, and capers.

Take: 500 mg of quercetin daily.

Medicinal Mushrooms

Medicinal mushrooms, used since ancient times to prevent and treat infection and disease, are also prized for their immunity-boosting power.

There are over 270 recognized species of medicinal mushrooms that are known to have immune-enhancing effects, including cordy-ceps, lion's mane, maitake, shiitake, reishi, and turkey tail; all have been shown to benefit the immune system. For instance, cordyceps, a traditional Chinese mushroom that produces various biopharmaceu-tical effects, was given to thirty-nine participants in a double-blinded study to see if the mushrooms enhanced their natural killer (NK) cells, a type of white blood cells found in the immune system. The study, published in the journal *BMC Complementary Medicine and Therapies*, found a significant enhancement in the activities of the NK cells.

To learn which medicinal mushrooms are available in your area, ask at your local health food store.

CHAPTER 19

Exercise to Strengthen Immunity

Exercise not only keeps your body in shape and is a great stress reliever, but it also has a profound effect on your immune system.

Research shows that performing regular moderate to vigorous exercise improves immune response, lowers chronic inflammation, and improves markers for a number of different diseases, including high blood pressure, obesity, and diabetes, those conditions that make people easy prey for COVID-19.

There is also plenty of research that shows that exercise helps bolster the immune system against many other viral infections, including influenza, rhinovirus (another cause of the common cold), and herpesviruses such as Epstein-Barr (EBV), varicella zoster (VZV), and herpes simplex virus 1 (HSV-1).

Even a daily walk helps prevent heart disease, high blood pressure, diabetes, obesity, and chronic obstructive pulmonary disease (COPD), the underlying risk factors for COVID-19. Exercise can also help prevent several different types of cancer, as well as strengthen survivors.

In addition, exercise has a profound effect in helping relieve symptoms of stress, which has been an enormous problem in the pandemic due to the threat to health, isolation, feelings of confinement, and worries about the economic toll. Even when the pandemic is over, these feelings are likely to linger.

The government's Physical Activity Guidelines for Americans recommend 150 to 300 minutes of moderate-intensity aerobic physical activity and two sessions per week of muscle strength training.

But even before the pandemic, more than 80 percent of Americans didn't meet these guidelines, the President's Council on Sports,

Fitness and Nutrition said, and then came the big shutdown, when fitness clubs, pools, beaches, and parks were closed and amateur sports games canceled.

Whether you are reading this during the pandemic or restrictions have eased or even lifted, it is always of paramount importance to have a strategy to make sure you get physical exercise, no matter the circumstances.

Here are suggestions from the American College of Sports Medicine on how to exercise during times when you must stay indoors or outdoors in small spaces when a COVID-19 spread is curbing your activities.

Aerobic Activities

- Put some music on and walk briskly around the house or up and down stairs for ten to twenty-five minutes, two to three times a day.
- Dance to your favorite music.
- Jump rope (if your joints can handle it).
- Do an exercise video. (You'll find lots of choices on the internet.)
- Use home cardio machines if you have them.
- Walk or jog around your neighborhood, staying six feet away from others.

Strength Training

- Download a strength workout app to your smartphone, such as the seven-minute workout.
- Do a strength training video.
- Do squats or sit-to-stands from a sturdy chair.
- Do push-ups against a wall, the kitchen counter, or the floor.
- Do lunges or single-leg step-ups on stairs.

CHAPTER 20

Ways to Reduce Stress

It's a known medical fact that after national disasters, such as hurricanes, earthquakes, and others, the heart attack rate spikes. So it's not unreasonable to expect this will occur after the pandemic, which has exacted an enormous toll on both our emotional health and our economic well-being.

This is because to deal with extreme stress, our minds fall back on a mechanism called the "flight or fight response."

Our bodies release a burst of hormones that prepare us to either run or fight, like our ancient ancestors would have if they were faced with, say, a charging saber-tooth tiger.

The hormones released are most notably adrenalin, which gives our heart rate and blood pressure a boost, and cortisol, which is a type of corticosteroid that suppresses the effectiveness of the immune system, inhibiting our ability to fight off antigens, which are substances on the surface of the cells. When this happens, our ability to fight off infection is decreased.

So here are ten easy ways for reducing stress, making your life more satisfying, and keeping your immune system strong as well:

1. Cut down on your TV news viewing. While we all need to stay informed, the all-news channels play events like the pandemic and other crises 24/7. Limit your news cycle to thirty to sixty minutes a day.

2. Plant a garden. Tending your own fruits and vegetables not only provides an excellent incentive to eat healthier but helps reduce stress as well. If you're pressed for space, you can grow

herbs in containers or find out if there is a community garden in your area.

3. Dance. When you engage in physical movement, like dancing, you release endorphins, the "happy hormones" that reduce stress. But if you have underlying health issues, remember to check with your doctor before starting any exercise workout, including dancing.

4. Sing. Another activity proven to release endorphins is singing. Church choirs and other concert groups offered opportunities for singing in public, but since singing is a "spreader" until the pandemic ends, you can sing at home or in the shower. Or put on some music. Even the act of listening to music has a proven uplifting and calming effect.

5. Unclutter your space. For many people, living in a cluttered environment is conducive to stress. Set out to clean only one room, not the whole house at once.

6. Do volunteer work. The act of volunteering and helping others less fortunate can not only reduce stress but also add purpose to life.

7. Cultivate forgotten interests. Did you formerly play bridge? Or paint? Go birdwatching or take photographs? Adult coloring has become a craze for stress reduction. Take a class or buy some supplies and let your imagination take over.

8. Take a stress-reduction course—many are offered online. As the country opens up, you can find them at community colleges, parks and recreation departments, or the local YMCA.

9. Reframe negative thoughts and practice positive thinking. Research suggests that anxiety, fear, and other negative states can affect the immune system.

10. Connect with your religious background. No matter what your religious denomination, your local church or synagogue is an excellent source of support. Your local church has the tools to help center your life. "Reading the Bible daily for me in this pandemic has been a great stress reducer for me and my family," Dr. Crandall notes.

The pandemic will likely turn out to be among the most memorable—and also one of the most stressful—events in our lives, given its impact on health, the economy, and the anxiety and isolation some of us have experienced.

If you are experiencing one or more of the stress indicators below, you might consider seeking professional help:

- fear and worry about your own health and the health of your loved ones
- depression
- changes in sleep or eating patterns
- difficulty sleeping or concentrating
- worsening of chronic health problems
- worsening of mental health conditions
- increased use of alcohol, tobacco, or other drugs

For anyone who feels they can't cope, the Centers for Disease Control and Prevention (CDC) recommends calling the Disaster Distress Helpline at 800-985-5990 to connect with a trained counselor. This is a toll-free, multilingual, and confidential crisis support service.

PART FOUR

Treating and Protecting against COVID-19

CHAPTER 21

How Severe COVID-19 Is Treated

For most COVID-19 patients, their cases start out mild, which is what happened to Joe. One night, as he was watching a TV show about the pandemic, he brushed his hair off his forehead and suddenly realized, "My forehead is on fire." But he put the thought out of his mind because he felt fine and had no other symptoms.

When COVID-19 symptoms worsen, most do so in five to ten days. Joe's worsened a little sooner—the following night. Still with a fever but feeling fine, he went to bed. When he awakened, it was fourteen hours later, his sheets were covered in sweat, he was shivering, and his teeth were chattering. He lay on the bed, shivering and feeling worn out.

His friend, a nurse practitioner, took him to the hospital, but as this was New York and the hospitals were overrun with COVID-19 patients, he was sent home. He got worse, so they went back to the hospital, and by the time they got there, to Joe, the room was spinning, and he kept fainting. They admitted him.

"I've never been that sick in my life," Joe recalls. His heart went into atrial fibrillation, a potentially deadly irregular heartbeat; his oxygen level fell; and he recalls spending a "brutal three days" in the hospital with an oxygen mask on his face. But he recalls, "I was lucky. The disease never went into my lungs." Joe spent several days in the hospital, suffering severe symptoms, but his condition gradually improved, and finally, he was discharged.

He was lucky. For many patients who develop serious complications, the virus gets into their lungs and they develop pneumonia. But it's not the usual kind of pneumonia, it's "COVID pneumonia," and it's different, says Dr. Richard Levitan, an emergency room doctor who volunteered to work in a New York City hospital during the pandemic.

Since COVID-19 is a brand-new ailment, doctors acknowledge that they are writing the playbook as they go along, trying different techniques to save patients' lives.

Pneumonia is a lung infection that causes inflammation in the tiny air sacs inside the lungs. They may fill up with fluid and pus, making it difficult to breathe.

But with COVID pneumonia, patients usually seem perfectly comfortable, possibly even chatting until it is suddenly realized that they have developed a shockingly low oxygen level—so severe that they need to be put on a ventilator, says Levitan, who urges doctors to evaluate patients with the use of an inexpensive pulse oximeter. This small device, placed on a patient's finger, provides an oxygen reading and can warn when the level falls dangerously low, even when patients don't realize it, which is what happens too often with COVID-19. (Earlier in this book, we noted that you can buy one of these devices as well, so you can monitor your oxygen level if you develop symptoms.)

The problem with pneumonia is that often it progresses to acute respiratory distress syndrome (ARDS), the same condition that kills patients who have influenza and other diseases.

In order to save them, they are put on ventilators, machines that essentially breathe for them. Ventilators do not provide any curative treatment; they buy time until patients recover on their own. But ventilators have a shockingly high mortality rate, especially when used for COVID-19.

According to a study done in the United Kingdom, of 3,883 patients with COVID-19 who were placed on ventilators, two-thirds, or 66.3 percent, died. This was much higher compared to the 35.1 percent for patients who require ventilation for regular viral pneumonia, the study, published in *Medscape* this past April, said. The reason isn't clear, experts say.

But when it comes to COVID-19, doctors are trying to improve on this poor survival rate, and one new technique they are using to save patients on ventilators is flipping them over on their stomachs, which is called "prone positioning." Seven years ago, French doctors published a study in the *New England Journal of Medicine* showing that patients with ARDS had a better chance of surviving if placed on their stomachs, and ever since, that method has been used in the United States to varying degrees, according to an article on CNN Health.

With the mortality rate for ventilated COVID-19 patients so high, some are wondering whether ventilators are the right way to go at all. In April, a medical team at Northwestern University used a machine called an extracorporeal membrane oxygenation (ECMO) machine to save the life of a patient with COVID-19.

The device is used to treat patients whose heart or lungs aren't working properly. It removes blood from the patient's body, pumps oxygen into the blood, then pumps the blood back into the body, according to physicians.

The device is used to relieve pressure on a sick patient's heart or lungs, and for the first time, it has been used to save the life of a patient fighting the coronavirus.

After the procedure, the patient was placed back on the ventilator and is expected to make a full recovery, according to the report from Channel 5 in Chicago, the local NBC affiliate.

Generally, ECMO machines are used only in extreme cases, and there aren't that many of them; since 2008, the number of them in U.S. hospitals has doubled from 108 to 264.

In the meantime, other hospitals are experimenting with alternatives to ventilators and reporting success, like University of Chicago Medicine, which reported "remarkable success" with COVID-19 patients using high-flow nasal cannulas, or HFNCs, which are noninvasive nasal prongs that sit below the nostrils and blow large volumes of warm, humidified oxygen into the nose and lungs. And there are other ventilator alternatives as well, as doctors struggle to save the lives of severely ill COVID-19 patients.

CHAPTER 22

New Drugs to Treat COVID-19

There are very few drugs that work against a virus, so COVID-19 poses a horrific problem. This was a deadly virus to which humans had no immunity, and there was also no treatment, so this has set off a worldwide race to come up with medications that can treat it. There were at least seventy drugs under development and 1,028 clinical trials underway as of this writing; here is a roundup of some of the most promising.

Remember to always consult your doctor about any medications you are considering.

Hydroxychloroquine-Chloroquine: From Malaria to COVID-19

Plaquenil is a combination of two drugs (hydroxychloroquine and chloroquine phosphate), which received Food and Drug Administration (FDA) approval some fifty years ago to treat malaria, and hydroxychloroquine is also approved as a treatment for lupus and rheumatoid arthritis.

The drugs have been found to kill the virus in lab tests, and there were also additional small reports attesting to the drug combination's effectiveness. On March 16, researchers from China reported in *Bio-Science Trends* that over one hundred people who had been treated with chloroquine had less severe disease and shorter hospitalizations.

Also, French researchers reported in the *International Journal of Antimicrobial Agents* that the combination of hydroxychloroquine and azithromycin, an antibiotic, given to thirty-six patients, had significantly reduced the amount of virus in their bodies.

The FDA granted emergency authorization on March 28, enabling the drug to be given to hospitalized COVID-19 patients, but also noted a list of side effects, including the drug's potential to cause heart rhythm disturbances.

In a paper published in *Nature Medicine* on April 24, researchers at New York University wrote that of eighty-four patients treated with hydroxychloroquine and azithromycin, nine experienced changes in heart rhythm that would put them at risk for severe arrhythmia or sudden cardiac death. Based on that, the FDA limited widespread use of the drug, saying it should only be given in a hospital setting or in clinical studies.

However, interest remains high in hydroxychloroquine either singly or in combination with chloroquine or other drugs, and more studies are underway.

Novartis, the drug's manufacturer, is enrolling 440 patients in a study to be conducted at more than a dozen sites in the United States.

Enrollment is also underway for a major multisite study sponsored by the University of Washington on the use of hydroxychloroquine and azithromycin in patients with COVID-19, and a study using these drugs is also getting underway in a multisite trial sponsored by the University of Washington in Seattle.

Remdesivir: Ebola Drug Turned COVID-19 Fighter

The most recent drug to win FDA emergency approval is remdesivir, which was originally developed for the Ebola outbreak in 2013 but did not pan out. But because was already shown to be safe in human trials, this drug got a giant leap ahead after it proved effective in shortening hospitalization time for COVID-19 patients.

Here's how it works: The virus that causes COVID-19 is an RNA virus, which infects by making copies of itself. Remdesivir mimics adenosine, one of the four building blocks of RNA. When the virus infects a cell and starts making copies, remdesivir inserts itself into the viral genome instead of adenosine and essentially blocks the replication process, instantly stopping the virus.

Initially, Gilead, the drug maker, first made remdesivir available in Wuhan, where it received favorable reviews in anecdotal use. Then it was tried in the United States on the very first COVID-19 case reported here: a thirty-five-year-old man who had just returned from

China. He was given the drug, and within a day, he improved dramatically, his doctors said.

The man was among twelve patients treated with the drug between January 20 and February 5, 2020. All the patients survived, although researchers noted these were not randomized, controlled studies. (These are studies in which one group of patients take the drug and the other group is given a placebo, or inactive substance, so researchers can discern if any effect is actually due to the medication.)

After that, Gilead launched a study with the University of Chicago Medicine on 125 patients, 113 of whom were severely ill with COVID-19. A video discussion about the drug was leaked in which doctors were seen making favorable comments, but again, it was not a randomized study.

Remdesivir continued to do well in small, nonrandomized studies, with the exception of one, which was published in *The Lancet* just a few days before the FDA's nod. That random controlled study found no difference between the drug and the placebo, although there were signs it might work if given earlier.

On April 29, the eagerly awaited results of a major multisite randomized controlled study trial were released that led to the drug's approval.

This study, called ACTT, was sponsored by the National Institutes of Health and had begun on February 21. The researchers gave 1,063 patients seriously ill with COVID-19 either remdesivir or a placebo via transfusion; the results showed that the drug reduced hospitalization by 31 percent, translating into an eleven-day hospital stay versus fifteen days for those who got the placebo. Since the results were based on interim data, no further details have yet been released.

Given the desperate need for the drug, the FDA granted emergency authorization, which was announced by President Trump in a White House ceremony with Vice President Pence, the FDA commissioner, and Gilead's CEO looking on.

There are caveats, though. First, emergency authorization enables doctors to give the drug to patients hospitalized with COVID-19 even though the drug has not been formally approved by the agency. This means that as of now, there is still no FDA-approved treatment for COVID-19.

Second, according to the FDA, the drug can cause liver damage, so patients must be checked daily. The regulatory agency also notes that remdesivir has not been given to that many patients, so there may be side effects yet to be discovered.

This isn't the game changer that everyone is hoping for. While the drug does shorten hospitalization, which is important, it does not affect a patient's likelihood of dying from COVID-19.

Regeneron Antibody Cocktail

Regeneron, which is repurposing an arthritis drug for use in COVID-19, is also the company behind an innovative plan to create a medication that both is a treatment for virus sufferers and also provides passive immunity to those who have not been infected, giving them a short-term vaccine-like protection against the disease.

Regeneron's approach is to identify the most powerful antibodies that defeat the SARS-CoV-2 virus (COVID-19). They have done this in two ways. First, their scientists have isolated antibodies from humans who have recovered from COVID-19. The concept is that these antibodies likely enabled those who recovered to beat the virus.

Second, Regeneron also genetically altered mice that have human-like immune systems that are then exposed to proteins in coronavirus 19 with the goal of them creating antibodies to fight COVID-19.

From these two approaches, Regeneron hopes to identify two of the best and strongest antibodies, creating a "cocktail" drug that will be used as a prophylaxis-like vaccine for people who don't have the disease. The same cocktail will be administered to those who have the virus.

All coronaviruses have a cell surface protein called the spike protein, which, as noted earlier in this book, enables the virus to latch onto a cell in the body and infect it. Regeneron's coronavirus 19 antibodies will target the spike protein in an attempt to block the interaction of the virus with the host.

The company's goal is to find one treatment using just two of the most powerful antibodies it can find that would both treat COVID-19 and create protection against it as well, similar to the action of a vaccine.

Regeneron has a positive track record using such antibody treatments. In 2018, after the Ebola outbreak in the Democratic Republic of Congo, the company created a three-antibody cocktail. In that case, a preliminary study proved so successful that the trial was stopped early in order to get the drug to the Ebola patients sooner.

The study compared experimental medicines with Mapp Biopharmaceutical Inc.'s ZMapp, also a three-antibody cocktail, which was considered the standard of care after a previous trial suggested it may help reduce death rates.

The results of the Ebola trial, published in *New England Journal of Medicine*, are nothing short of breathtaking.

In the trial, 681 Ebola patients were administered three drug treatments, including Regeneron's antibody cocktail, ZMapp, and remdesivir, the widely hailed drug for COVID-19.

The trial was abruptly stopped after results demonstrated that Regeneron's antibody cocktail produced results far superior to ZMapp and Remdesivir.

After twenty-eight days on the Regeneron cocktail, 66.5 percent of patients survived compared to 48.7 percent for those on ZMapp. Remdesivir proved slightly better than ZMapp, with a mortality rate of 53 percent during the same period.

Most importantly, the study indicated that if the Regeneron drug is administered early, when viral loads are low, the survival rate after twenty-eight days jumps to almost 89 percent.

The company's drug plan has already received preliminary approval from the FDA, and they are expecting to begin clinical trials on humans in June 2020. If these trials prove positive, the Regeneron cocktail could be widely available by the fall of 2020.

Antigen Therapy: Using Patients' Blood to Protect Others

Although not yet approved by the FDA, doctors are already using blood from recovered COVID-19 patients to pass along their immunity to others who are fighting the disease.

This treatment, also called "convalescent plasma," has been in use for one hundred years in treating other types of viral illnesses, including measles, chickenpox, polio, and severe acute respiratory syndrome (SARS).

When your body is exposed to a foreign pathogen, such as a virus, the body's immune response is to produce antibodies, which are proteins that can bind to the virus and prevent it from invading the other cells in the body. Even after the threat from the invading virus is gone, these antibodies stay in the blood, protecting you from further infections.

For this treatment, the plasma, or liquid part of the blood, is collected from recovered patients and transfused into patients who are sick with COVID-19.

Earlier, two promising small studies on plasma in China had sparked enthusiasm for the treatment here. The first was a study from Shenzhen, China, published in the *Journal of the American Medical Association*, which detailed the plasma treatment given to five critically ill patients with acute respiratory distress syndrome (ARDS), a devastating end-stage condition of the disease.

After receiving the treatment, the amount of virus in the patients was reduced, and their conditions improved.

The second Chinese study, posted online, looked at ten critically ill patients and noted a marked improvement in their conditions after the treatment, including in seven, in whom the virus had completely disappeared.

These were small studies and not randomly controlled, but based on such results, the FDA, while not formally approving the technique, provides for its use in clinical trials and grants doctor's individual approval to use it in individual patients.

There are also large, randomized clinical trials getting underway in this country, including a $250 million study at Columbia University Mailman School of Public Health, sponsored by Amazon, and a three-hundred-patient study at NYU Langone Health, both in New York City.

A key problem is that no one knows how strong the antibodies from COVID-19 are or how long they will last to fight infection. But thousands of patients who have recovered from COVID-19 are already clamoring to donate their plasma, so this pandemic may be a golden opportunity to see if this type of therapy indeed does work.

Famotidine: Repurposed Heartburn Drug under Study

Among the long list of drugs under testing is a familiar name—Pepcid. The active ingredient for the over-the-counter heartburn medication is indeed being tested as a treatment for COVID-19, only at nine times the dosage and administered intravenously.

Interest in the drug was sparked when an adventurous infectious disease specialist, Michael Callahan, had gone to Wuhan, China, on an avian flu project around the time the COVID-19 epidemic began to explode according to the journal, *Science*.

The virus was killing one out of five patients over the age of eighty, but Callahan's attention was drawn to a group of survivors who happened to be poor.

In reviewing 6,212 of their records, he noticed that many of them suffered from chronic heartburn, for which they were taking famotidine, or Pepcid, instead of the more expensive drug of choice, omeprazole, or Prilosec.

Hospitalized COVID-19 patients on famotidine appeared to be dying at a rate of about 14 percent compared with 27 percent for those not on the drug, although this result was not significant.

The records were far from peer-reviewed studies, but they intrigued Callahan, and he brought them to Robert Kadlec, an assistant secretary at the Department of Health and Human Services, and also to Robert Malone, chief medical officer of Alchem Laboratories, which is headed by Malone. Malone also is involved in a sophisticated project that focuses on FDA-approved drugs that can be repurposed.

After getting FDA-approval for a study, the U.S. Biomedical Advanced Research and Development Authority (BARDA), which operates under Kadlec, gave Alchem a $20.7 million contract for the trial.

Although it hasn't been proven to work on COVID-19 yet, here is an explanation of one theory on why it might.

Famotidine is in a class of medications called H2 blockers, and it works by decreasing the amount of acid made in the stomach.

Prescription famotidine is typically used to treat ulcers, gastro-esophageal reflux disease, and other conditions where the stomach produces too much acid.

It's thought that the drug, when given in far higher dosages than currently sold, may bind to a viral enzyme (protease), which enables the virus to multiply.

To find out, enrollment is currently underway by New York City's Northwell Health, which is aiming to recruit 1,175 people to learn if the main ingredient of a common heartburn drug will turn out to be a game changer in the treatment of COVID-19.

Ivermectin: Can a Head Lice Killer Treat COVID-19?

Both old and new drugs are being eyed in the race to find a treatment for COVID-19, and among them is ivermectin, a familiar antiparasitic treatment for head lice and scabies.

As noted previously, FDA-approved drugs are enticing prospects for drug makers because these medications already have proven safety records, and ivermectin is no exception.

Discovered in the late 1970s, ivermectin, which originated in the soil of Japan, was originally a veterinary drug used to kill a wide range of parasites, both internal and external, in animals. Dubbed a "wonder drug," like aspirin, it was later discovered to have a multitude of uses for human ailments, including head lice, scabies, river blindness (onchocerciasis), roundworms, whipworm, and more.

Ivermectin is now being touted as a COVID-19 treatment by the Victorian Infectious Diseases Reference Laboratory (VIDRL) and Monash University, both located in Melbourne, Australia.

A new study, published in the journal *Antiviral Research*, has found that ivermectin knocked out coronavirus 19 with a single dose in lab cultures.

The investigators infected cell cultures with isolates from coronavirus 19 and then treated them with ivermectin. The drug removed all signs of the virus within forty-eight hours.

This Australian study caught the interest of clinical investigators from Medincell, a French pharmaceutical research venture adjacent to Montpellier. As it turns out, this group had received a $6.4 million grant from Unitaid, a global health initiative that is supported by the foundation headed by Bill Gates and his wife, Melinda.

Now the French venture has launched a research initiative to develop a long-acting injectable version of ivermectin and plans to embark on a clinical study in the hopes of creating an effective and affordable way to help control the global COVID-19 pandemic.

Repurposing HIV Drugs to Treat COVID-19

The global HIV drug market is expected to grow from $27 billion in 2019 to about $30.5 billion in 2020 due to an increase in demand for such drugs for the treatment of COVID-19 patients, according to a May report in Business Wire.

Currently, several countries—including the United States—are evaluating antiviral drugs used to treat HIV, the virus that causes AIDS, eyeing their use on COVID-19.

The HIV drugs ritonavir and lopinavir (sold as a combination therapy by AbbVie under the brand name Kaletra) have been tested against COVID-19 in clinical trials, but with mixed results.

In Wuhan, China, at the peak of the COVID-19 epidemic, 199 adults, with a median age of fifty-eight, hospitalized with severe complications from the virus were randomized to receive ritonavir and lopinavir (LPVr). After twenty-eight days, the results found no difference between the two groups, although the safety of the drug combination was proven and additional trials were planned to verify the results, according to the study, which was published in the *New England Journal of Medicine*.

However, LPVr is not the only HIV drug currently under study; another is the emtricitabine and tenofovir combination therapy known as Truvada, which is given as part of a drug regimen to HIV patients to suppress the virus by blocking its replication. It is similar to remdesivir, discussed earlier as the drug that received emergency FDA authorization in May, but it can be given orally, as opposed to remdesivir, which requires intravenous injection.

Researchers in Spain became curious about Truvada after seeing relatively few HIV-positive people develop severe complications from COVID-19, so they launched a study that aims to enroll four thousand participants and will be randomized into groups in which some will be given Truvada; some will be given hydroxychloroquine, the antimalarial drug mentioned earlier; and some will receive both medications together.

Once the study is complete, researchers will assess whether any of the regimens lowered the number of symptomatic COVID-19 cases or reduced the severity of the disease, the researchers said.

Stem Cell Treatment: Mobilizing the Immune System against COVID-19

One of the most innovative ways to fight COVID-19 is a method that uses stem cells to mobilize the immune system and galvanize them to block COVID-19 from taking over the body's cells.

Dr. Robert Hariri, a surgeon, biomedical scientist, and a successful engineer, heads Celularity, a New Jersey–based company that is pioneering the effort.

The cell therapy works by boosting the body's early immune response in a way that could target the coronavirus.

The company transforms placental stem cells into one-size-fits-all "natural killer" (NK) cells, which are a type of lymphocyte (white blood cell), which is a component of the immune system.

When the coronavirus invades the body, the immune system tries to hunt down the intruder, but the virus is able to initially disable it. These stem cells would act as guards to keep the virus from getting out of control while giving the immune system time to mount a response and knock it out.

Stem cells are special human cells that are able to develop into many different cell types, ranging from muscle cells to brain cells.

Celularity is awaiting the start of a clinical trial.

The company had originally developed the stem cell technique as a cutting-edge cancer treatment but believes its technology is transferable to COVID-19.

But there are those who question whether this therapy will work. Viruses and NK cells are familiar to each other, so there is a concern the virus will be able to evade the NK cells.

Another concern is that boosting the immune response could inadvertently ignite the "cytokine storm" response that is so deadly in COVID-19 patients.

CHAPTER 23

When Will There Be a Vaccine?

Experts agree that we will be vulnerable to COVID-19 until a vaccine against it is developed.

Vaccines contain the same germs that cause disease, but they have been either killed or weakened to the point that they don't make you sick.

A vaccine stimulates your immune system to produce antibodies, exactly as it would if you were exposed to the disease. After getting vaccinated, you develop immunity to that disease without having to get the disease first.

Developing a vaccine is a time-consuming and arduous process that can take fifteen to eighteen years if started from scratch. This is because, since a vaccine is intended for healthy people, it would have to undergo a round of safety testing first, followed by a large clinical trial in which the vaccine is administered to people along with a control group, who would receive an inactive substance, and sufficient time would need to pass to determine whether or not it was effective.

In addition, any vaccine that is approved would have to be manufactured in amounts large enough to provide coverage to protect the country, also a time-consuming task.

But with numerous teams of scientists throughout the world racing to develop a vaccine, this time frame is expected to quicken considerably. Some global consortiums already working together so that separate initiatives are not duplicated.

There are no vaccines for coronaviruses, but there are some factors that could give this one a head start. First, scientists already have the complete genome for this virus, which could help in the development of both treatments and a vaccine.

In addition, scientists can take advantage of work already underway on the development of a vaccine for the other two known coronaviruses, severe acute respiratory syndrome (SARS) and Middle East respiratory syndrome (MERS), which are related to coronavirus 19.

The MERS vaccine is still under development, but that virus is primarily contained in the Arab peninsula, and since SARS disappeared, a vaccine is no longer needed. (No one fully understands why SARS vanished, but this could have been due to social distancing, experts say.)

One problem that could arise in terms of virus development is that like other coronaviruses, as well as the flu, these viruses tend to mutate, which makes finding an effective vaccine difficult and is why the flu vaccine must be given each year. Every year, scientists predict which flu virus strains will be circulating and then create a vaccine based on their best predictions, which is what some believe will happen with coronavirus 19.

But one top virologist and technology investor is much more optimistic when it comes to a time frame. Peter Kolchinsky, the cofounder of the Boston-based RA Capital Investment, believes in a faster timetable, predicting a vaccine could come as soon as this fall.

This timetable is "ambitious and aggressive," he acknowledges, and he agrees that if problems arise, it will probably take an additional year.

There are more than sixty vaccines now under development, the World Health Organization (WHO) says. Here's a look at some promising ones.

Oxford University

In the race to develop a vaccine, scientists at Oxford University in the United Kingdom are among those leading, having already begun human trials of a coronavirus vaccine they hope to have ready by fall.

The scientists at Jenner University had a head start because their vaccine is a version of one they had already proved in trials of similar inoculations that were harmless to humans, the *New York Times* notes.

The vaccine, which has shown promise in rhesus monkeys, is made up of a weakened version of the common cold virus (called an adenovirus) but is genetically altered to make it "impossible" to grow in humans. They have combined this adenovirus with genes that code for the coronavirus (spike) protein that the virus uses to infect human cells. They hope that by using this vaccination, the body will recognize and mount an immune response to the coronavirus protein that will stop the virus from entering the body's cells.

They are involved in recruiting more than six thousand people, hoping to show that not only is the vaccine safe, but it is also effective.

Johnson & Johnson

Johnson & Johnson, in a landmark partnership with the U.S. Department of Health and Human Services, along with other companies, is developing a vaccine, and they are pledging to supply one billion doses for worldwide use during the pandemic.

The company expects to initiate human trials of a vaccine by September and anticipates the first batches of the COVID-19 vaccine would be ready for an emergency-use authorization by early next year.

Like other drug makers, Johnson & Johnson is tapping into the knowledge it used to develop its experimental Ebola virus vaccine, which was used in the outbreak in the Democratic Republic of Congo, along with the work it has done with Zika and HIV.

Sinovac Biotech

Also in the race is the Chinese drug maker Sinovac Biotech, the first company to market a vaccine for swine flu, which says it's now in the position to start producing one hundred million units a year.

Dubbed "Coronavac," the experimental vaccine entered human trials at the end of April, and although it has far to go, the company says it already has thousands of doses ready to go.

Like Oxford University, Sinovac is also using rhesus monkeys to test its vaccine, which is an old-fashioned formulation consisting of a chemically inactivated version of the virus. Earlier in April, Sinovac said it had demonstrated that it had protected eight rhesus monkeys from COVID-19.

CHAPTER 24

Antibody Testing

As noted earlier, coronavirus tests break into two broad categories. Diagnostic tests check for the virus to see if you are currently infected with COVID-19.

Antibody tests look to see if you were infected in the past and recovered, which means you may have built up an immune response that could offer you some protection from becoming infected again.

Here is how antibodies work.

Also known as immunoglobulins, antibodies are Y-shaped proteins produced by the body's immune system to help stop intruders from harming the body. When an intruder, like a virus, enters the body, the immune system springs into action.

There are two ways in which the U.S. population will develop immunity against COVID-19—through a vaccine or through "herd immunity."

Herd immunity is a form of indirect protection from an infectious disease that occurs when a large population has contracted the illness and built up an immune response.

But building herd immunity against a virus as infectious as the coronavirus may take a while, according to the World Health Organization (WHO).

In the early days of the coronavirus' spread, scientists from the WHO estimated the infectious rate of the coronavirus was 2.2 compared to that of seasonal flu, which stands at 1.28. But with more research, they recently revised that ranking upward to 5.7, according to research published in the journal *Emerging Infectious Diseases*.

Here's why that's important: if the ranking of the coronavirus had stayed at 2.2, it would mean that only about 55 percent of our population would have to become immune by becoming infected and recovering before the pathogen ran out of people to infect.

But at an infectious rate of 5.7, this means that 85 percent of the population needs to become immune before health officials can be confident that there will not be a second wave of infections.

When the pandemic hit, some countries, like the United Kingdom, experimented with herd immunity but had to backpedal when deaths began to mount. But there is also a concern that by using restrictions like social distancing, we may be keeping people from becoming infected but delaying herd immunity, which, in essence, could make it take longer to see the end of COVID-19.

What about Sweden?

One country that is sticking to herd immunity is Sweden, which has issued some restrictions but has basically chosen to allow the virus to spread, with mixed results.

People are encouraged to work from home, nursing homes are closed, and universities have moved to online learning. But on the other hand, public schools are still open, as are restaurants, bars, and gyms, although some social distancing is in place.

But Sweden has paid a price; as of late April, they had 16,755 confirmed cases of COVID-19 and 2,021 deaths, a large portion of them the elderly. In contrast, neighboring Norway and Denmark, which took more stringent measures, have just a fraction of those numbers.

But as with everything else about coronavirus 19, there tend to be more questions than answers.

Are Antibody Tests Accurate?

There have been two problems with antibody tests—getting enough of them and their accuracy. Originally in short supply, the test supply situation is improving now, but there are still questions about accuracy. One recent study showed they can have a false positive rate of up to 15 percent. This means that up to 15 percent of the time, people will be told they have the antibodies to COVID-19 and may have built up some immunity, but they actually haven't. Companies are working to improve on the accuracy of these tests.

Once You've Had COVID-19, Can You Get It Again?

No one knows the exact answer to that question. Most scientists believe that once you recover from COVID-19, you will be initially protected, although it's not yet known how strong that immunity is or how long it lasts.

Once You Recover from COVID-19, Can You Still Give the Disease to Someone Else?

No, but you still need to wait a little bit before leaving quarantine. According to the Centers for Disease Control and Prevention (CDC), you are no longer infectious if you've been free of fever for seventy-two hours without the use of fever-reducing medicine. (Bear in mind that recent studies show that not everyone with COVID-19 gets a fever.) You should also have recovered from any respiratory symptoms, and this should be at least seven days since the onset of symptoms, the CDC says.

The test-based strategy that the CDC suggests involves getting negative results on two tests, with samples collected at least twenty-four hours apart.

Once You've Had COVID-19, Are You Immune for Life?

Again, no. When it comes to viruses, there are some cases where you are immune for life. This is true of measles, for instance. In the case of COVID-19, it may be that people are immune for a period of time—say, for a year—but will need to be revaccinated, as is done for the seasonal flu.

CHAPTER 25

Is COVID-19 Here to Stay?

During the pandemic, the world mobilized to get rid of coronavirus 19, but there were always unsettling indications that even when this is accomplished, COVID-19 may continue to be a threat.

Recently, Deborah Birx, the White House's coronavirus task force coordinator, said, even while state officials were expressing optimism that the coronavirus was dampening down and outlining plans to reopen their economies, that some form of the social distancing laws adopted during the panic would likely have to remain through the summer.

But will summer be enough? Many health officials, including Dr. Anthony Fauci, the country's top infectious disease expert, has declared, "We will have coronavirus in the fall. I am convinced of that."

Centers for Disease Control and Prevention (CDC) director Robert Redfield also concurs, predicting that the return of the coronavirus, coupled with the advent of the flu season, could place a disastrous strain on the nation's health system, especially considering that by April 21, the virus had already killed more than forty-two thousand people across the country.

In fact, not only have health officials warned of a second wave of COVID-19 hitting in the fall, when the weather gets cooler, but there is evidence that the virus may also become an unwelcome annual visitor, just like the flu.

According to an article on Biospace.com, four separate research groups working in the United States, Australia, and China analyzed the effect of temperature and humidity on the coronavirus. They predict that while hot summer temperatures and humidity could reduce the amount of virus, the coronavirus will likely return in the fall, when the humidity drops and temperatures cool down.

One of the groups, researchers from the Harvard T. H. Chan School of Public Health, looked at how two seasonal coronaviruses, beta coronaviruses OC43 and HKU1, operate. These are two common human coronaviruses that cause cold-like symptoms.

According to the team's simulation, infections with SARS-CoV-2 (COVID-19) might also become a seasonal occurrence, as is the case with the other beta coronaviruses that infect humans, they said in the journal *Science*.

"We should prepare for annual or sporadic outbreaks every few years," Stephen Kissler, a biomathematician and lead author of the study, told the *Wall Street Journal*.

But viruses don't always follow seasonal patterns, say other scientists, who have observed that the worse outbreaks of the Spanish flu in 1918–19 came during the summer.

Whatever happens, as the nation edges back to normalcy, health officials are warning that people should not forget the social distancing and other precautions learned during the pandemic, because these measures are likely to be needed until a vaccine is developed to protect against recurrent COVID-19.

CHAPTER 26

Protecting Loved Ones in Nursing Homes

One of the highest, most heartbreaking death tolls in the pandemic has been the number of most vulnerable who have died: the residents in our nation's nursing homes.

Because of their age, frailty, and underlying medical conditions, the residents in nursing homes became among the first in the United States to die, and these deaths have not stopped, resulting in some of the most horrific stories coming out of the pandemic.

Adding to the heartbreak is the fact that in order to try to contain the virus, these facilities almost from the start were shut off from visitors, including family members, who were left to worry.

At a time like a pandemic, you have to be proactive and make sure to ask questions constantly so that the nursing home knows that you are watching out for your elder family and friends, even from a distance.

Here is a list from AARP of things you should ask to make sure the facility your family members are in is being kept safe:

- Has anyone in the nursing home tested positive for COVID-19? This includes residents, staff, or other vendors who may have been in the nursing home.
- What is the nursing home doing to prevent infections?
- What precautions are taken for residents who are not in private rooms?
- Is the nursing home currently at full staffing level for nurses, aides, and other workers?

- How is the nursing home staff being screened for COVID-19, especially when they leave and reenter the building?
- Does the nursing home have personal protective equipment (PPE), such as masks, face shields, gowns, and gloves that they need to keep residents safe?
- What is the nursing home doing to help residents stay connected with their families or loved ones during this time?
- What is the plan for the nursing home to communicate important information to both residents and families on a regular basis?
- Will the nursing home be contacting you by phone or email, and when?
- What is the plan to make sure the needs of nursing home residents are met—such as bathing, feeding, medication management, and social engagement—if the nursing home has staffing shortages?

How to Ease Social Isolation

Your loved ones may or may not realize why you can no longer visit them. Here are some tips to help you keep in touch, even at a distance:

- Talk to your loved one using FaceTime or Google Duo or a similar app on your smartphone. If the person in the nursing home doesn't have a smartphone, an aide or nurse may be able to help.
- If you've set this up before you were shut out during the pandemic, make sure you make good use of Facebook's Portal, Google Nest Hub, or a similar type of device to make frequent virtual visits with your loved one.
- Digital photo frames are a way to send a multitude of photos that your loved one can look at while they are in the nursing home. You can make one at home and bring it to the nursing home office and ask them to deliver it; all the nurse or aide needs to do is plug it in and tap the power button to get it started.
- Don't forget that sending cards, actual photos, or flowers are also great ways to keep in touch and let your loved one know they are not forgotten.

- If you live nearby, ask if you can arrange to have your loved one brought to a window or door so that you can at least exchange a wave.
- Don't assume your loved one will remember why you aren't visiting. Always remind them that you want to, you love them, and you will see them as soon as you are able.

HOW TO CREATE
YOUR PERSONAL
COVID-19 STRATEGY

Now that society is reopening, it's critical for everyone to take personal responsibility to reduce exposure to COVID-19. The best way to stay safe is to think and plan ahead. Here is advice on how to create your personal COVID-19 strategy.

- Make sure your immune system is in top shape. Follow the guidelines in this book for sleep, diet, supplements, exercise, and reducing stress. Going out means encountering more opportunities for infection, so you'll want to give your body every advantage to fight back and win.
- Review our chapter on risk factors to figure out where you stand, in terms of your age and underlying medical conditions. You can use this as a guide to decide which activities pose the least risk for you.
- Track the spread. Contact your municipality and learn how to access their website that tracks COVID-19 cases. Which numbers to watch? Dr. Natasha Martin, an assistant medical professor of UC San Diego, who is leading the project to test all the students there, recommends watching hospitalizations. If the numbers are going up, cut back on your public activities.
- No matter where you want to go, like a restaurant, spa, retail store, etc., find out in advance what COVID-19 protections are being done, in terms of social distancing, masking, and disinfecting. If you're uneasy, chose another place, or don't go.
- Fresh air is better than indoors. If you have a choice of eating outside, or indoors, opt for an airy location, where the virus load will be lesser.
- Avoid large, crowded public gatherings, including concerts, auditoriums, athletic games, etc. Limit gatherings for the time being.

- Beware of hidden traps. Don't lick stamps, for instance, because the coronavirus can linger on envelopes. Going to the bank? Opt for the drive-through. Be meticulous about your personal cleanliness—short, clean nails are best. Avoid long fingernails, which can harbor a pathogen.
- Above all else, don't live your life in fear. COVID-19 is likely to be with us for a while. Stay alert and be careful, but always dwell in faith, secure in the knowledge that we will conquer this plague, just as we have triumphed over others that came before it. As said Jesus, "Don't be afraid, just believe."

*   *   *

Billy Graham has said:

"When we worry, anxiety about the future takes root in our minds and hearts, and we become more fearful and unsettled. Constant worry also leaves to doubt—doubt in ourselves, but most of all doubt in God and his Love for us. And yet worrying never changes anything."

ABOUT THE AUTHORS

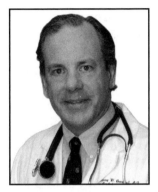 **Chauncey W. Crandall IV, M.D., F.A.C.C.,** is a renowned cardiologist in the United States and the leader of medical missions across the world for forty years, leading medical teams on the front lines of battle and waging a war against the plagues that devastate poor communities throughout the world.

He is Director of Preventive Medicine at the Palm Beach Cardiovascular Clinic and Chief of Interventional Cardiology at Good Samaritan Medical Center in Palm Beach, Florida.

His passion for heading to medical crises all over the world began early, when, at the age of nineteen, he traveled to the jungles of Africa and worked stateside with world-famous anthropologist Colin M. Turnbull. He gained early training in pandemics at Yale University, where he was introduced to Dr. Robert Gallo, the virologist who discovered the HIV virus that leads to AIDS.

Over his career, Dr. Crandall has performed over forty thousand heart procedures. He regularly lectures nationally and internationally on a variety of cardiology topics, and he is author of several top-selling health books, including *The Simple Heart Cure*, and he is the editor of the popular medical newsletter *Dr. Crandall's Heart Health Report*.

Dr. Crandall continues to devote much of his life's work to the poor, the suffering, and the dying and personally ministers to the sick in areas forgotten by others.

He has been heralded for his values and message of hope and victory that he brings to his patients in the United States and that he spreads to others throughout the world.

To contact Dr. Crandall:
Dr. Chauncey Crandall
c/o Chadwick Foundation
P.O. Box 3046
Palm Beach, FL 33480
chaunceycrandall.com

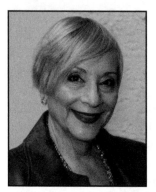

Charlotte Libov is an award-winning health book author and a health reporter with expertise in pandemic outbreaks.

She is a heart disease survivor whose experience with open-heart surgery inspired her first book, *The Women's Heart Book*, which was one of the first to raise the issue of heart disease in women.

Her books include *The Cancer Survival Guide* (American Society of Journalism and Authors' "Self Help Book of the Year"), *A Women's Guide to Heart Attack Recovery*, and *Beat Your Risk Factors*, among others.

She has appeared on TV and radio shows across the country. A popular speaker, she has given talks for Toyota, IBM, the Biotechnology International Convention, the American Heart Association, Duke University, and the U.S. Army War College, as well as many other hospital systems, health organizations, and schools around the country.

Her byline has appeared regularly in *Newsmax Magazine*, Newsmax Health.com, WebMD.com, CURE.com, AARP.com, GoodHousekeeping .com, and many other websites and publications. She is a former regular contributing writer to the *New York Times* and a managing editor of *Neurology Now*.

Her passion for fighting COVID-19 stems from one of her aunts, who tragically contracted the Spanish flu as a child and was left a lifelong invalid.

To contact Charlotte Libov:
Email: sobechar@gmail.com
www.libov.com

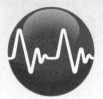
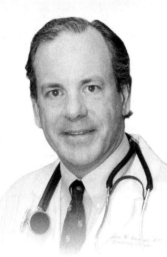

More Titles From Humanix Books You May Be Interested In:

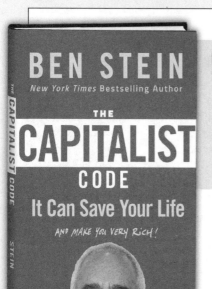

Warren Buffett says:

"My friend, Ben Stein, has written a short book that tells you everything you need to know about investing (and in words you can understand). Follow Ben's advice and you will do far better than almost all investors (and I include pension funds, universities and the super-rich) who pay high fees to advisors."

In his entertaining and informative style that has captivated generations, beloved *New York Times* bestselling author, actor, and financial expert Ben Stein sets the record straight about capitalism in the United States — it is not the "rigged system" young people are led to believe.

Dr. Mehmet Oz says:

"*SNAP!* shows that personalities can be changed from what our genes or early childhood would have ordained. Invest the 30 days."

New York Times bestselling author Dr. Gary Small's breakthrough plan to improve your personality for a better life! As you read *SNAP!* you will gain a better understanding of who you are now, how others see you, and which aspects of yourself you'd like to change. You will acquire the tools you need to change your personality in just one month — it won't take years of psychotherapy, self-exploration, or re-hashing every single bad thing that's ever happened to you.

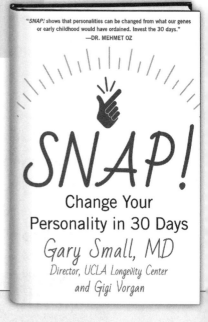

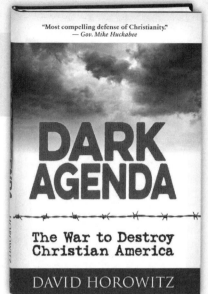
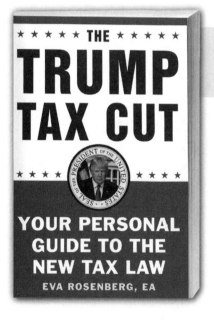

Is Your Immune System Ready?

Make Sure Your Immune System Is Strong, to Combat Any Viruses, Germs or Bacteria!

Your Immune System Weakens with Age!

By midlife, the bone marrow produces fewer stem cells to develop into immune-enhancing cells.

The thymus gland shrinks, reducing immune T-cells. And worn-out immune cells accumulate, leading to an imbalanced inflammatory process.

Immune function is further diminished with aging by a number of factors, including stress, diet, poor sleep, lack of exercise, pollution, and many others.

To counteract the many challenges to the aging immune system, holistic physician Dr. David Brownstein, M.D., formulated the advanced immune support formula **RETAMIN®** — with 9 powerful ingredients.

Wellmune® Boosts Key Immune Responses

As the flagship ingredient in **RETAMIN**, patented Wellmune® strengthens natural body defenses without overstimulating the immune system.

Nine double-blind, placebo-controlled human clinical studies show it mobilizes key immune cells to protect against the harmful effects of physical, emotional, and lifestyle stress.

Best of all, Wellmune begins to provide immune support within 1 to 2 days — and is safe and effective for people of all ages.

In addition to Wellmune, **RETAMIN** contains 8 more hard-working ingredients:

Maitake Mushrooms. Contain beta glucans for immune defense.

Olive Leaf Extract. This helps balance the inflammatory process, crucial for optimal immune function.

Zinc. This trace mineral helps maintain a healthy thymus in aging individuals. The thymus gland is important in immune health.

Astragalus. This adaptogenic herb helps defend the body against physical, mental, and emotional stress.

Vitamin D. Helps stimulate immune cell production and the secretion of important compounds called immunoglobulins. Older adults are at increased risk of vitamin D insufficiency.

Vitamins A, C, and E. These immune health superstars play key roles in immunity and in the body's antioxidant defense system. Vitamins C and E also help maintain a balanced inflammatory response.

As you can see, **RETAMIN** is not a simple one-ingredient nutrient. **RETAMIN** has made it easy to help support robust immune health — no matter your age. Try **RETAMIN** today!

Medix Select can send you a 30-day trial supply of **RETAMIN** to try for yourself. Simply cover a $4.95 shipping charge and enroll in our convenient Smart Ship program.

Learn More: Retamin.com/Book

These products are not intended to diagnose, prevent, treat, or cure any disease. Always consult with a physician before using these or any such products.